Clinical
Laboratory
Safety

Susan L. Rose,
MT(ASCP), MS, DA

Health Scientist
U.S. Department of Energy
Washington, DC

Clinical
Laboratory
Safety

VNR VAN NOSTRAND REINHOLD
New York

Printed in the United States of America

Van Nostrand Reinhold
115 Fifth Avenue
New York, New York 10003

Van Nostrand Reinhold International Company Limited
11 New Fetter Lane
London EC4P 4EE, England

Van Nostrand Reinhold
480 La Trobe Street
Melbourne, Victoria 3000, Australia

Nelson Canada
1120 Birchmount Road
Scarborough, Ontario M1K 5G4, Canada

16 15 14 13 12 11 10 9 8 7 6 5 4 3 2

Library of Congress Cataloging-in-Publication Data

Rose, Susan L.
  Clinical laboratory safety.

  Bibliography: p.
  Includes index.
  1. Medical laboratories — Safety measures. I. Title. [DNLM: 1. Laboratories
— Standards — United States.   2. Accident prevention.   QY 23 R797c]
R860.R67 1984   616.07′56′0289   83-9923
ISBN 0-397-50615-5

It is with love that I dedicate this book to

My mother, Clara Rose, Greg and Edie Harper, and my dear little nephew, Scott, for being the sunshine in my life;

My brand new niece, Rebecca, for being something wonderful to look forward to;

My Aunt Florence and Uncle Steve Levitas for always being there no matter what my needs;

Carolyn Moser, for the best in friendship, caring, and typing—a great combination;

And not lastly, my dearest friend Paul for all his hugs, invincibility, and smiles.

Foreword

Hospital laboratories are a critical part of health care, for it is there that data essential to the proper diagnosis and care of patients are discovered. One of the important lessons of recent history is that as new information about health and disease comes forth from the research community, health care becomes even more dependent on the hospital laboratory.

We are fortunate to be living in the midst of a true revolution in our understanding of human biology. The future for increased understanding of health and disease is brighter than ever before. Hence, the serious and important functions of the laboratory are emphasized as never before.

Persons working in hospital and other clinical laboratories are vital to high-quality care. As such, they must be well informed on all aspects of the operation of the laboratory. This includes adherence to a mandatory set of safe operating procedures, adequate knowledge of potential laboratory hazards, and familiarity with the significant safety regulations with which they must comply. Dr. Rose has written a book that explains these in readable form. *Clinical Laboratory Safety* is complete in its coverage, and its contents should be known and understood by everyone who works in the laboratory setting.

The successful operation of hospital laboratories is essential to the proper care of patients, and the contents of this book are vital to the successful operation of laboratories.

EDWARD N. BRANDT, JR., M.D.
Assistant Secretary for Health
U.S. Department of Health and Human Services
Washington, DC

Preface

As clinical laboratory analyses have become more numerous and varied and complex instrumentation has become further integrated into all aspects of the laboratory, so have knowledge and pervasiveness of laboratory occupational hazards increased. Until now, there has been no single resource to supply the kinds of safety information essential to the well-being of the entire laboratory staff. Common sense alone no longer adequately protects the employee in a modern hospital-based clinical laboratory. Safety training and education are essential but educational materials are, at best, fragmentary; they are usually borrowed unaltered from other disciplines, frequently dependent on a time-consuming literature search, or often available only in a multimedia approach necessitating the use of audiovisual equipment. With the publication of *Clinical Laboratory Safety,* this information gap no longer exists.

The objective of this book, to provide an original, comprehensive, and easily read text, is achieved by exploring fully the hazards that may be encountered in the clinical laboratory and then supplying the detailed methods and actions necessary to assure occupational safety of the personnel. The text begins by examining the legal basis of health and safety concerns for the worker—the federal Occupational Safety and Health Act of 1970 and then addresses other regulatory and accrediting agencies as they relate to laboratory safety. Each of the major laboratory departments is covered separately so that unique hazards can be identified and methods of control enumerated for that particular area. Ubiquitous hazards such as hepatitis virus are referred to in several sections, as appropriate. The individual laboratory discussions (Chap. 2–6) are followed by Chapter 7, Fire, Compressed Gases, and Electricity—safety concerns in *all* clinical laboratory departments. In Chapter 8, accidents, emergency planning, assignment of responsibilities, safety equipment, and a short first-aid discussion are presented, also from the perspective of the entire laboratory.

In Chapter 9, the book concludes with a comprehensive, yet fairly explicit, discussion of laboratory waste. This material, again relevant to all departments, is intended to raise the level of awareness of every laboratory professional, indicate the serious nature of careless waste disposal, and provide a rational approach to this growing problem in and for the laboratory.

Throughout the text, somewhat dramatic narrative is used to capture the reader's attention and to illustrate the severity of the hazards encountered. Original photographs, tables, and figures are used to provide simplification of concepts and clarity of meaning.

SUSAN L. ROSE, MT(ASCP), MS, DA

Acknowledgments

The great lesson I learned while writing this book is that people are really wonderful to a stranger with a request for help. Every time I called on people with a request or a question, they responded with answers, written material, further contacts, encouragement, and often friendship. As a result, adequate thank-yous would certainly fill another book, so I will limit myself here to a very few of the wonderful people who came to my aid on this project. Several of these people were friends of mine to begin with, but an incredible number more will have become friends as a result of this book. This gift alone has made the entire effort worthwhile.

My acknowledgments are random and no part of the list is secondary to any other. The list is, however, very incomplete.

Lisa Biello, Darlene Pedersen, and Barbara Farabaugh, Editors, J. B. Lippincott Company, Philadelphia, PA

Dr. Edward Brandt, U.S. Department of Health and Human Services, Washington, DC

Dr. Eugene Kennedy and Dr. Barbara J. Howard, Catholic University of America, Washington, DC

Dr. John Fox and the laboratory staff at Providence Hospital, Washington, DC

Dr. Vernon Martens, Michele Best, and the laboratory staff at Washington Hospital Center, Washington, DC

Camille Atwood, Norfolk General Hospital, Norfolk, VA

Dr. J. W. Thiessen, Carolyn Moser, and Dr. Joseph Blair (ret), U.S. Department of Energy, Washington, DC

Mr. David Slade, Small Affairs Photography, Silver
Spring, MD

Deanna Duby and Bernadette Wiermanski, A.S.C.P.,
Washington, DC

Adrienne Weller, Gordon Briggs, and Frances Ryan,
C.A.P., Washington, DC and Skokie, IL

Arthur Gass and Lillie Clark, OSHA, Washington, DC

Claire Welty, Environmental Protection Agency, Washington, DC

Dr. John Forney, Office of Laboratory Improvement,
Centers for Disease Control, Atlanta, GA

Dr. Gene Del Polito, A.S.M.T., Washington, DC

Marie Cameron, Children's Hospital National Medical
Center, Washington, DC

Milton Anderson, Bureau of Laboratories, Department
of Human Services, Washington, DC

Bill Argonza, Laboratory Field Services, California State
Department of Health, Berkeley, CA

Gordon McKinnon, Editor, National Fire Protection
Association, Quincy, MA

Sallie Tyrrell, Merck Sharp and Dohme, West Point, PA

Kent Weber and W. Norton, J. T. Baker Chemical Company, Phillipsburg, NJ

Barbara Tucker, Safety Director, Abbott Northwest
Hospital, Minneapolis, MN

Dr. Robertson Augustine, John Leach, Monica Schaeffer,
and Agnes Richardson, Division of Safety, National
Institutes of Health, Bethesda, MD

Mary Halbert, School of Public Health, University of
Minnesota, Minneapolis, MN

Joan Logue, National Commission for Clinical Laboratory Standards, Villanova, PA

The laboratory photographs were taken at Providence Hospital
and Washington Hospital Center, Washington, DC, with permission of
the pathologists, Drs. John Fox and Vernon Martens respectively. Dave
Slade of Silver Spring, Maryland, was the photographer.

Contents

1

A Regulatory Overview

The following example of a serious accident could happen in *any* hospital laboratory—even yours!

It was not a routine day for one medical technician in the Clinical Center. A request for more space had finally been approved and the physical chore of moving chemicals and other supplies into a new laboratory had to begin. The chore was made more pleasant for the technician by the prospect of putting things exactly where she wanted them, choosing shelf heights, and having everything finally within easy reach.

Her first task was to adjust the shelves along one wall. She then squatted down to view the new spacing. To test the fit, she reached behind where she sat for one of the full glass gallon bottles of concentrated sulfuric acid she had so carefully transported from the old laboratory. Suddenly, the technician was awash in a flood of slippery sulfuric acid and broken glass. Her pensive mood immediately gave way to sheer panic and helplessness. As she tried to free herself from the burning acid, she fell and knocked over another full bottle of sulfuric acid. Now, no longer squatting, she lay directly in the fuming acid.

Her screams of terror brought help quickly from next door. A colleague ran in and saw the broken glass, the spilled acid, and the hysterical technician. When he reached out to help her, she inadvertently resisted, splashing acid on the would-be rescuer as well. Nonetheless, he dragged her out into the hall, pulling against her resistance and getting himself further burned in the process. When he finally got her under the safety shower in the hall, he released her and reached out to pull the safety ring, drenching them both in water. He continued to pull the ring, rinsing away the acid, which clung stubbornly to their skin and clothes. A second person arrived to help. With large laboratory shears, the rescuer rapidly cut away the clothes of the sopping wet, shocked technician, who sat dazed under the showering spray. Luckily, she had been clad in shoes, jeans, and a laboratory coat, which minimized the severity of the initial acid burns to her legs and feet. However, because of the large volume of acid spilled and the way she fell, she did sustain second- and third-degree burns to her thighs and buttocks. She was taken to the emergency room for treatment of shock and burns. Although she did survive the accident, the technician required a long hospital stay and ultimately needed plastic surgery to repair the damage to her skin. The two rescuers did exactly as they should have. They removed the victim as rapidly as possible from the area, showered her with water, did not try to neutralize the acid on her skin, and cut away her acid-soaked clothes.

This was one of the worst accidents the Clinical Center had ever had, but it is surely not unique among the nation's hospital laboratories. Ask almost any experienced medical technologist and he can relate at least one such horror story—a compressed-gas cylinder hurtling itself through a wall, a sodium-azide explosion in the laboratory drain, a shattered culture of live tuberculosis (TB) aerosol floating out of the centrifuge into the air, and on and on . . .

True, some of these past experiences probably should no longer occur because new laws and regulations outlaw certain chemicals and procedures in the laboratory. Bear in mind, however, that the modern hospital laboratory is routinely a highly technical workplace with very hazardous chemicals, complex electronic instruments, and a wide variety of pathogens. To keep the laboratory a safe, accident-free place to learn and to practice the highly technical skills demanded of each laboratory professional requires a sound knowledge of the potential hazards, an understanding of the standard safety procedures to which one must adhere, and a constant vigilance and concern for safety. To aid in maintaining this safe environment for you and your co-workers, this manual was written. It is for *your* safety that it must be read and used.

A formidable array of rules, standards, and regulations set forth by federal, state, and local agencies and professional organizations demand, as far as possible, safe and healthful working conditions in the hospital laboratory. Working toward the elimination of hazards and the use of safe laboratory procedures is not just a sensible goal—it is the *law!* To proceed in any other manner is, therefore, not an option.

Although complete freedom from danger, risk, or injury is incompatible with the laboratory function and mission, adequate knowledge of workplace hazards provides the margin of occupational safety required by law.

A comprehensive knowledge of the subject of laboratory safety requires an overview of the relevant organizations, regulations and policies (see Definitions on page 4). Let us begin at the federal level.

The U.S. Constitution (and, in parallel fashion, the state constitutions) grants Congress the authority to pass laws and to create agencies and departments to protect and promote public health and welfare. These departments and agencies in turn can and *must* establish rules and regulations to carry out the law. This "fine tuning" by the agencies allow them more flexibility and greater control in writing the standards and regulations than they would have if Congress itself wrote them all. The agencies seek public comment, knowledgeable peer groups, and other specialists to aid them in formulating the regulations. The agencies are also able to revise regulations in a more timely manner than the rewriting of a law by Congress would allow. The flexibility, however, complicates matters for laboratory personnel, who must comply with a vast and changing body of rules and regulations. Further compounding the difficulty of seemingly continuous updating are the court decisions, administrative-board decisions, and official interpretations that may effectively modify any law or regulation. Nonetheless, it is the responsibility of the laboratory staff to remain informed and in compliance at all times. Once rules are made, they must be enforced. This legal authority is exercised by investigations, inspections, granting of licenses, variances and permits, judicial determinations, certification, reciprocity with other organizations, and even exemptions and exclusions.

REGULATORY OVERVIEW—DEFINITIONS

Accreditation A voluntary process recognized as a measure of quality. It is used by some regulatory agencies as one criterion for granting certification and licensure. Standards for accreditation may be similar or identical to standards for licensure. Accrediting organizations are usually based on peer approval, voluntary quality control, education, and consultation.

Certification or **Licensure** Regulatory measures of a facility's ability to operate.

Licensure The process by which an agency or government grants permission to persons or facilities, meeting predetermined qualifications, to engage in a given occupation, use a particular title, or perform specified functions.

Certification The process by which a nongovernment agency or association grants recognition to a person who has met certain predetermined qualifications specified by that agency or association.

Equivalency or **Reciprocity** A mechanism for comparing programs and functions so that one may be used in lieu of the other. Often the legal body (*e.g.,* a federal agency) maintains authority and stringency over standards even when another organization is deemed (identified as) an acceptable or equivalent alternative authority.

Guideline Suggested operating practice or procedure often broadly written, that can be modified or used as written. Use of guidelines may be voluntary and is often established by the private sector to self-govern its activities.

Inspections Careful, critical, on-the-scene examinations that determine violations against an accepted or legal standard. Inspections may be for accreditation, licensure, certification, or safety. Depending on the inspection type, it may or may not be announced ahead of time.

Law A rule, passed by a legislative authority, often written in broad, general language. An agency designated by the law will establish or promulgate the specific regulations.

Regulation The specific details by which a law may be implemented. Proposed regulations appear in the *Federal Register* prior to final adoption, so that interested groups may comment.

Standards Specific criteria, to be used unmodified for materials, methods, or practices. Use of a standard may be voluntary or mandatory depending on whether it is put forth by a voluntary-consensus standard-setting group or a government agency (see Appendix E for professional standard-setting groups.)

FEDERAL AND NONFEDERAL AGENCIES AND LAWS CONCERNED WITH SAFETY

Now that the regulatory process has been introduced, we will examine the federal laws and the agencies themselves, beginning with the landmark worker-safety legislation—the Occupational Safety and Health Act (OSHA) of 1970.

Occupational Safety and Health Act (OSHA)

In 1970, Congress sought to establish uniform and comprehensive protection against safety and health hazards in the workplace. Statistics compiled for that year showed 14,000 worker deaths, 2.5 million worker disabilities, and 300,000 new incidences of occupational diseases (see *All About OSHA*, a publication of the U.S. Department of Labor). The cost and burden were staggering and the incidence was increasing. Therefore, in 1970 the U.S. Congress passed OSHA, which promised to ". . . assure so far as possible every working man and woman in the Nation safe and healthful working conditions and preserve our human resources." According to the Act, this would be accomplished through the following:

1. By encouraging employers and employees in their efforts to re-duce the number of occupational safety and health hazards at their places of employment, and to stimulate employers and em-ployees to institute new and to perfect existing programs for pro-viding safe and healthful working conditions;
2. By providing that employers and employees have separate but independent responsibilities and rights with respect to achieving safe and healthful working conditions;
3. By authorizing the Secretary of Labor to set mandatory occupa-tional safety and health standards applicable to businesses affect-ing interstate commerce, and by recreating an Occupational Safety and Health Review Commission for carrying out adjudica-tory functions under the Act;
4. By building upon advances already made through employer and employee initiative for providing safe and healthful working con-ditions;
5. By providing for research in the field of occupational safety and

health, including the psychological factors involved, and by developing innovative methods, techniques, and approaches for dealing with occupational safety and health problems;

6. By exploring ways to discover latent diseases, establishing causal connections between diseases and work in environmental conditions, conducting other research relating to health problems, in recognition of the fact that occupational health standards present problems often different from those involved in occupational safety;

7. By providing medical criteria which will assure insofar as practicable that no employee will suffer diminished health, functional capacity, or life expectancy as a result of his work experience;

8. By providing for training programs to increase the number and competence of personnel engaged in the field of occupational safety and health;

9. By providing for the development and promulgation of occupational safety and health standards;

10. By providing an effective enforcement program which shall include a prohibition against giving advance notice of any inspection and sanctions for any individual violating this prohibition;

11. By encouraging the states to assume the fullest responsibility for the administration and enforcement of their occupational safety and health laws by providing grants to the states to assist in identifying their needs and responsibilities in the area of occupational safety and health, to develop plans in accordance with the provisions of this Act, to improve the administration and enforcement of state occupational safety and health laws, and to conduct experimental and demonstration projects in connection therewith;

12. By providing for appropriate reporting procedures with respect to occupational safety and health which procedures will help achieve the objectives of this Act and accurately describe the nature of the occupational safety and health problem;

13. By encouraging joint labor–management efforts to reduce injuries and disease arising out of employment.

The following overview presents, in brief, provisions of the Occupational Safety and Health Act that have relevance to the clinical laboratorian.

Agencies Created by the Act

Two new Federal agencies were created in 1970 by OSHA. They are the National Institute for Occupational Safety and Health (NIOSH) and the Occupational Safety and Health Administration (OSHA).* Brief mission statements that follow provide an introduction to these agencies. (See field locations for OSHA and regional offices for NIOSH for the addresses of the regional offices for each; if more detailed information is desired, the regional offices should be contacted.)

NIOSH is one of eight operating components of the Centers for Disease Control (CDC). The CDC, itself a health agency in the Department of Health and Human Services, is discussed in a later section. NIOSH is the primary federal agency engaged in research to eliminate on-the-job hazards to the health and safety of America's workers. NIOSH is responsible for identifying occupational safety and health hazards, for developing measures to control them, and for recommending federal standards to limit the hazards. When requested by an employer or employees, NIOSH conducts health-hazard evaluations of workplaces. NIOSH also has a manpower training program designed to help alleviate the critical shortage of occupational safety and health personnel. NIOSH does *not* regulate, issue, or enforce safety or health standards. This function is carried out by OSHA.

OSHA, within the Department of Labor, promulgates and enforces safety and health standards and regulations in the workplace. It also conducts workplace investigations and inspections to determine the status of compliance with job safety and health standards. When noncompliance with safety and health regulations and standards is found, OSHA issues citations and proposes penalties.

Laboratory Coverage

All hospital laboratories (and their employees), except federal, state, and municipal hospital laboratories, are covered directly under OSHA. Executive Order 12196 (1980) makes federal agencies themselves (*e.g.,* Department of Energy, Environmental Protection Agency) subject to OSHA, and as a result each is required to maintain safety and

(Text continues on p. 12)

*Note that OSHA may be used to refer to either the Occupational Safety and Health Administration or the Occupational Safety and Health Act of 1970.

OCCUPATIONAL SAFETY AND HEALTH ADMINISTRATION (OSHA) FIELD LOCATIONS

Region I
(Connecticut, Maine, Massachusetts, New Hampshire, Rhode Island, Vermont)
16–18 North Street
1 Dock Square Building, 4th floor
Government Center
Boston, MA 02109
(617) 223-6710
FTS 223-6710

Region II
(New York, New Jersey, Puerto Rico, Virgin Islands, Canal Zone)
Room 3445 (1 Astor Plaza)
1515 Broadway
New York, NY 10036
(212) 944-3426
FTS 265-3426

Region III
(Delaware, District of Columbia, Maryland, Pennsylvania, Virginia, West Virginia)
Gateway Building, Suite 2100
3535 Market Street
Philadelphia, PA 19104
(215) 596-1201
FTS 596-1201

Region IV
(Alabama, Florida, Georgia, Kentucky, Mississippi, North Carolina, South Carolina, Tennessee)
1375 Peachtree Street, N.E.
Suite 587
Atlanta, GA 30367
(404) 881-3573
FTS 257-3573 or 2281

Region V
(Illinois, Indiana, Minnesota, Michigan, Ohio, Wisconsin)
230 South Dearborn Street
32nd Floor, Room 3244
Chicago, IL 60604
(312) 353-2220
FTS 353-2220

Region VI
(Arkansas, Louisiana, New Mexico, Oklahoma, Texas)
555 Griffin Square, Room 602
Dallas, TX 75202
(214) 767-4731
FTS 729-4731

Region VII
(Iowa, Kansas, Missouri, Nebraska)
911 Walnut Street, Room 406
Kansas City, MO 64106
(816) 374-5861
FTS 758-5861

Region VIII
(Colorado, Montana, North Dakota, South Dakota, Utah, Wyoming)
Federal Building, Room 1554
1961 Stout Street
Denver, CO 80294
(303) 837-3061
FTS 327-3061

Region IX
(California, Arizona, Nevada, Hawaii, Guam, American Samoa, Trust Territory of the Pacific Islands)
11349 Federal Building
450 Golden Gate Avenue
Box 36017
San Francisco, CA 94102
(415) 556-0586
FTS 556-0586

Region X
(Alaska, Idaho, Oregon, Washington)
Federal Office Building
Room 6003
909 First Avenue
Seattle, WA 98174
(206) 442-5930
FTS 399-5930

NATIONAL INSTITUTE FOR OCCUPATIONAL SAFETY AND HEALTH (NIOSH) REGIONAL OFFICES

Region I
(Connecticut, Maine, Massachusetts, New Hampshire, Rhode Island, Vermont)
DHHS, Region I
Government center (JFK Federal Building)
Boston, MA 02203
(617) 223-6668
FTS 223-6668

Region II
(New Jersey, New York, Puerto Rico, Virgin Islands)
DHHS, Region II—Federal Building
26 Federal Plaza
New York, NY 10275
(212) 264-2485
FTS 264-2485

Region III
(Delaware, District of Columbia, Maryland, Pennsylvania, Virginia, West Virginia)
DHHS, Region III
P.O. Box 13716
Philadelphia, PA 19101
(215) 596-6716
FTS 596-6718

Region IV
(Alabama, Florida, Georgia, Kentucky, Mississippi, North Carolina, South Carolina, Tennessee)
DHHS, Region IV, Division of Preventive Health Services
101 Marietta Tower, Suite 1007
Atlanta, GA 30323
(404) 221-2396
FTS 242-2396

Region V
(Illinois, Indiana, Michigan, Minnesota, Ohio, Wisconsin)
DHHS, Region V
300 South Wacker Drive, 33rd Floor
Chicago, IL 60606
(312) 886-3881
FTS 886-3881

Region VI
(Arkansas, Louisiana, New Mexico, Oklahoma, Texas)
DHHS, Region VI
1200 Main Tower Building, Room 1835
Dallas, TX 75202
(214) 767-3916
FTS 729-3916

Region VII
(Iowa, Kansas, Missouri, Nebraska)
DHHS, Region VII
601 East 12th Street, 5th Floor West
Kansas City, MO 64106
(816) 374-5332
FTS 758-5332

Region VIII
(Colorado, Montana, Utah, Wyoming, North Dakota, South Dakota)
DHHS/PHS/PREVENTION—Region VIII
1194 Federal Office Building
Denver, CO 80294
(303) 837-3979
FTS 327-3979

Region IX
(Arizona, California, Hawaii, Nevada, Guam)
DHHS, Region IX
50 United Nations Plaza
San Francisco, CA 94102
(415) 556-3781
FTS 556-3781

Region X
(Alaska, Idaho, Oregon, Washington)
DHHS, Region X
1321 Second Avenue (Arcade Plaza Building)
Seattle, WA 98101
(206) 442-0530
FTS 399-0530

health programs consistent with the OSHA standards for private employers. OSHA provisions do *not* apply to state and local governments as employers except in state-plan or agreement states that have explicitly included them.

Laboratory Standards

OSHA states that each employer must provide a place of employment that is "free from recognized hazards that cause or are likely to cause death or serious harm to employees." It also makes OSHA responsible for "promulgating legally enforceable standards, which may require conditions or adoption or use of one or more practices, means, methods, or processes reasonably necessary to protect workers on the job." Employers have a responsibility to become familiar with the standards applicable to their laboratories and to ensure that their employees have and use personal protective gear and equipment as required. When there are *no* specific standards, employers are responsible for adhering to the intent of the Act's general duty clause, which states in effect that a safe and healthy workplace must be provided for employees. Obviously, safety hazards that are not anticipated by regulations can and do occur. In these instances, the compliance officer may cite the general duty clause as a legal reference to require removal of the hazard or issue a violation.

OSHA standards for the safety and health of all workplaces fall into four major categories: General Industry, Maritime, Construction, and Agriculture. Clinical, chemical, and analytic laboratories are subject to the relevant standards found within *OSHA General Industry Standards and Interpretations, Volume 1,* Part 1910, Title 29 Code of Federal Regulations (OSHA 29 CFR 1910 [available as OSHA Publication 2206]). The subject index to these standards appears in Appendix A.

The General Industry Standard addresses a broad range of health and safety requirements such as adequate lighting, noise control, electrical and fire safety, warning and exit signs, medical examinations, and exposures to toxic substances. The clinical laboratory can and must comply with those regulations that apply. However, the section on Exposure to Toxic and Hazardous Substances (Subpart Z) was written for manufacturing and industrial exposures and therefore has been challenged as inappropriate for clinical, academic, and research laboratories, where exposures are small or nonexistent and employees are professionals trained to work safely with chemicals. Efforts are underway to remedy this situation and to promulgate a standard designed for laboratories. Information on the status of Subpart Z with respect to the clinical laboratory may be obtained from the Department of Labor, OSHA Health Standards Programs. The address is as follows:

Health Standards Programs
U.S. Department of Labor
Occupational Safety and Health Administration
200 Constitution Avenue, N.W.
Washington, DC 20210

When a new standard (Subpart Z) is approved, every effort will be made to inform the affected laboratories (see Appendix A).

Laboratory administrative and supervisory personnel should be familiar with OSHA 29 CFR 1910 and all other regulations that may affect their facilities. When federal standards of any sort are to be changed, the proposed modifications are printed in the *Federal Register*, which is available from the Superintendent of Documents, U.S. Government Printing Office (GPO), Washington, DC 20402. Each year all currently in-effect regulations and standards are published in the Code of Federal Regulations (CFR), also available from the GPO.

Standards development may begin on recommendations or petitions from employers, employees, standard-setting organizations, advisory committees, NIOSH petitions, or an OSHA initiative. The planned, revoked, new, or revised standards appear in the *Federal Register* and public comment is solicited. After a comment period, a final standard and effective date are published, along with reasons (given in a preamble) for implementing the standards. For various reasons, employers may be granted a variance, or exception, to the standard, allowing some flexibility in the application of the law.

Recordkeeping and Reporting

Employers of 11 or more employees must maintain records of all injuries and illnesses as they occur. An occupational injury is any injury resulting from a work-related accident or exposure involving a single incident in the laboratory. An occupational illness is any abnormal condition or disorder caused by exposure to environmental factors associated with employment.

Recordable injuries are those resulting in death, lost workdays, restriction of work, loss of consciousness, job transfer, or medical treatment other than first aid. On-the-job accidents resulting in an employee death or hospitalization of five or more employees must be reported to the nearest OSHA office. Recordkeeping forms are maintained on a calendar-year basis and must be available for five years at the worksite (Figs. 1-1 and 1-2). A copy of the last page of the OSHA workplace injury and illness log must be posted annually, during the month of February, in each laboratory.

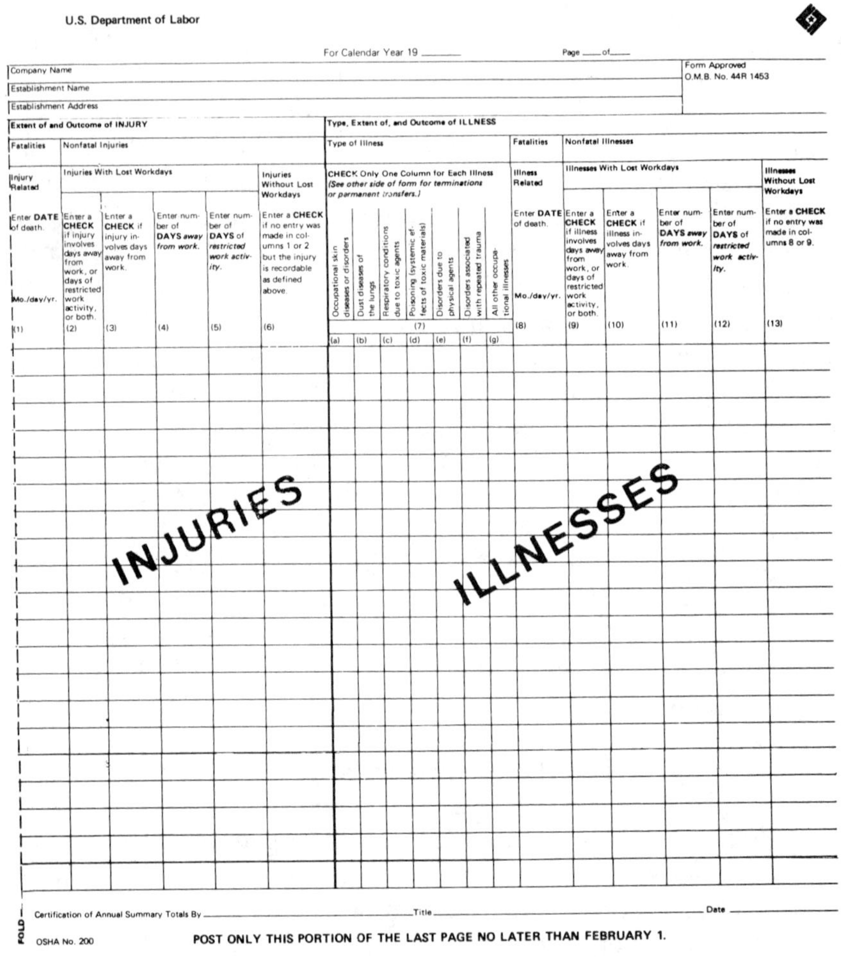
U.S. Department of Labor

For Calendar Year 19 ____ Page ___ of ___

Company Name

Establishment Name

Establishment Address

Form Approved O.M.B. No. 44R 1453

Extent of and Outcome of INJURY

Fatalities — Injury Related — Enter **DATE** of death. Mo./day/yr. (1)

Nonfatal Injuries — Injuries With Lost Workdays:
- (2) Enter a **CHECK** if injury involves days away from work, or days of restricted work activity, or both.
- (3) Enter a **CHECK** if injury involves days away from work.
- (4) Enter number of **DAYS** *away from work.*
- (5) Enter number of **DAYS** of *restricted work activity.*

Injuries Without Lost Workdays — (6) Enter a **CHECK** if no entry was made in columns 1 or 2 but the injury is recordable as defined above.

Type, Extent of, and Outcome of ILLNESS

Type of Illness — **CHECK** Only One Column for Each Illness *(See other side of form for terminations or permanent transfers.)* (7)
- (a) Occupational skin diseases or disorders
- (b) Dust diseases of the lungs
- (c) Respiratory conditions due to toxic agents
- (d) Poisoning (systemic effects of toxic materials)
- (e) Disorders due to physical agents
- (f) Disorders associated with repeated trauma
- (g) All other occupational illnesses

Fatalities — Illness Related — Enter **DATE** of death. Mo./day/yr. (8)

Nonfatal Illnesses — Illnesses With Lost Workdays:
- (9) Enter a **CHECK** if illness involves days away from work, or days of restricted work activity, or both.
- (10) Enter a **CHECK** if illness involves days away from work.
- (11) Enter number of **DAYS** *away from work.*
- (12) Enter number of **DAYS** of *restricted work activity.*

Illnesses Without Lost Workdays — (13) Enter a **CHECK** if no entry was made in columns 8 or 9.

INJURIES

ILLNESSES

Certification of Annual Summary Totals By ____ Title ____ Date ____

FOLD

OSHA No. 200 POST ONLY THIS PORTION OF THE LAST PAGE NO LATER THAN FEBRUARY 1.

Fig. 1-1. OSHA Form 200. Record of occupational injuries and illnesses.

OSHA No. 101
Case or File No. _____

Form approved
OMB No. 44R 1453

Supplementary Record of Occupational Injuries and Illnesses

EMPLOYER

1. Name _____

2. Mail address _____
     (No. and street)   (City or town)   (State)

3. Location, if different from mail address _____

INJURED OR ILL EMPLOYEE

4. Name _____ Social Security No. _____
   (First name)   (Middle name) (Last name)

5. Home address _____
     (No. and street)   (City or town) (State)

6. Age _____ 7. Sex: Male_____ Female_____ (Check one)

8. Occupation _____
     (Enter regular job title, *not* the specific activity he was performing at time of injury.)

9. Department _____
     (Enter name of department or division in which the injured person is regularly employed, even
     though he may have been temporarily working in another department at the time of injury.)

THE ACCIDENT OR EXPOSURE TO OCCUPATIONAL ILLNESS

10. Place of accident or exposure _____
     (No. and street)   (City or town)   (State)
  If accident or exposure occurred on employer's premises, give address of plant or establishment in which
  it occurred. Do not indicate department or division within the plant or establishment. If accident occurred outside employer's premises at an identifiable address, give that address. If it occurred on a public highway or at any other place which cannot be identified by number and street, please provide place
  references locating the place of injury as accurately as possible.

11. Was place of accident or exposure on employer's premises? _____ (Yes or No)

12. What was the employee doing when injured? _____
          (Be specific. If he was using tools or equipment or handling material,
_____
     name them and tell what he was doing with them.)
_____

13. How did the accident occur? _____
     (Describe fully the events which resulted in the injury or occupational illness. Tell what
_____
happened and how it happened. Name any objects or substances involved and tell how they were involved. Give
_____
full details on all factors which led or contributed to the accident. Use separate sheet for additional space.)

OCCUPATIONAL INJURY OR OCCUPATIONAL ILLNESS

14. Describe the injury or illness in detail and indicate the part of body affected. _____
          (e.g.: amputation of right index finger
_____
     at second joint; fracture of ribs; lead poisoning; dermatitis of left hand, etc.)

15. Name the object or substance which directly injured the employee. (For example, the machine or thing
  he struck against or which struck him; the vapor or poison he inhaled or swallowed; the chemical or radiation which irritated his skin; or in cases of strains, hernias, etc., the thing he was lifting, pulling, etc.)
_____
_____

16. Date of injury or initial diagnosis of occupational illness _____
          (Date)

17. Did employee die? _____ (Yes or No)

OTHER

18. Name and address of physician _____

19. If hospitalized, name and address of hospital _____
_____

  Date of report _____ Prepared by _____
  Official position _____

Fig. 1-2. OSHA Form 101. Supplementary record of occupational injuries and illnesses.

OSHA is now experimenting with various ways to reduce the paperwork burden in those industries with good safety records and low risk of injury. Regional OSHA administrators can provide the local requirements for participation to interested laboratories.

Employee Information

Each laboratory must have the following posted in a prominent location:

- The OSHA workplace poster (Fig. 1-3)
- Summary of petitions for variance
- Copies of OSHA citations for violation of standards
- Log and summary of injuries and illnesses (Fig. 1-1)

Employees exposed to toxic substances have a right to see their medical-examination and exposure records and have a right to know the toxic or hazardous compounds that they are exposed to or that are used in the facility. Information such as the Material Safety Data Sheet (see Fig. 3-3) for the various chemicals used should be accessible to all employees.

Inspections

Every laboratory covered under the Act is subject to inspection by OSHA compliance safety and health officers. An employee representative has a right to accompany the compliance officer during an inspection. Employees also have the right to talk privately with the inspector and to identify hazards or describe accidents.

Employees may request an OSHA inspection or a NIOSH hazards evaluation of their workplace. The requesting employee's name will be kept confidential by both agencies. In no case under the terms of the OSHA Section 11C may an employee who has identified a hazard or complained to OSHA or NIOSH be punished by the employer. Inspections begin with the locations providing the most serious physical or health hazards. The inspections include employer and employee consultations, recordkeeping examinations, and a thorough inspection of the laboratory.

Citations may be issued at or following the inspection, and penalties of up to $10,000 may be imposed for each violation. In extreme

job safety and health protection

The Occupational Safety and Health Act of 1970 provides job safety and health protection for workers through the promotion of safe and healthful working conditions throughout the Nation. Requirements of the Act include the following:

Employers: Each employer shall furnish to each of his employees employment and a place of employment free from recognized hazards that are causing or are likely to cause death or serious harm to his employees; and shall comply with occupational safety and health standards issued under the Act.

Employees: Each employee shall comply with all occupational safety and health standards, rules, regulations and orders issued under the Act that apply to his own actions and conduct on the job.

The Occupational Safety and Health Administration (OSHA) of the Department of Labor has the primary responsibility for administering the Act. OSHA issues occupational safety and health standards, and its Compliance Safety and Health Officers conduct jobsite inspections to ensure compliance with the Act.

Inspection: The Act requires that a representative of the employer and a representative authorized by the employees be given an opportunity to accompany the OSHA inspector for the purpose of aiding the inspection.

Where there is no authorized employee representative, the OSHA Compliance Officer must consult with a reasonable number of employees concerning safety and health conditions in the workplace.

Complaint: Employees or their representatives have the right to file a complaint with the nearest OSHA office requesting an inspection if they believe unsafe or unhealthful conditions exist in their workplace. OSHA will withhold, on request, names of employees complaining.

The Act provides that employees may not be discharged or discriminated against in any way for filing safety and health complaints or otherwise exercising their rights under the Act.

An employee who believes he has been discriminated against may file a complaint with the nearest OSHA office within 30 days of the alleged discrimination.

Citation: If upon inspection OSHA believes an employer has violated the Act, a citation alleging such violations will be issued to the employer. Each citation will specify a time period within which the alleged violation must be corrected.

The OSHA citation must be prominently displayed at or near the place of alleged violation for three days, or until it is corrected, whichever is later, to warn employees of dangers that may exist there.

Proposed Penalty: The Act provides for mandatory penalties against employers of up to $1,000 for each serious violation and for optional penalties of up to $1,000 for each nonserious violation. Penalties of up to $1,000 per day may be proposed for failure to correct violations within the proposed time period. Also, any employer who willfully or repeatedly violates the Act may be assessed penalties of up to $10,000 for each such violation.

Criminal penalties are also provided for in the Act. Any willful violation resulting in death of an employee, upon conviction, is punishable by a fine of not more than $10,000 or by imprisonment for not more than six months, or by both. Conviction of an employer after a first conviction doubles these maximum penalties.

Voluntary Activity: While providing penalties for violations, the Act also encourages efforts by labor and management, before an OSHA inspection, to reduce injuries and illnesses arising out of employment.

The Department of Labor encourages employers and employees to reduce workplace hazards voluntarily and to develop and improve safety and health programs in all workplaces and industries.

Such cooperative action would initially focus on the identification and elimination of hazards that could cause death, injury, or illness to employees and supervisors. There are many public and private organizations that can provide information and assistance in this effort, if requested.

More Information: Additional information and copies of the Act, specific OSHA safety and health standards, and other applicable regulations may be obtained from your employer or from the nearest OSHA Regional Office in the following locations:

**Atlanta, Georgia
Boston, Massachusetts
Chicago, Illinois
Dallas, Texas
Denver, Colorado
Kansas City, Missouri
New York, New York
Philadelphia, Pennsylvania
San Francisco, California
Seattle, Washington**

Telephone numbers for these offices, and additional Area Office locations, are listed in the telephone directory under the United States Department of Labor in the United States Government listing.

Washington, D.C.
1981
OSHA 2203

Raymond J. Donovan

Raymond J. Donovan
Secretary of Labor

U. S. Department of Labor
Occupational Safety and Health Administration

GPO 878-195

Fig. 1-3. The OSHA workplace poster.

cases (*i.e.,* assaulting a compliance officer) criminal penalties may be imposed.

A system of legal appeals and review is established to carry out this process in a fair manner. The Occupational Safety and Health Review Commission, an independent executive board, hears contested cases. Its decisions may be appealed to federal appellate courts.

OSHA-Approved State Programs

The Act allows and encourages states to develop and operate their own safety and health programs. To be approved, any state plan must provide for the development and enforcement of safety and health standards that are, or will be, at least as effective as standards set forth under OSHA. Once a plan is approved, OSHA will fund 50% of the state program operating costs. By 1982, 22 states, Puerto Rico, and the Virgin Islands had OSHA-approved state plans. OSHA continues to monitor state plans once they are approved. In some cases, state plans cover only public-sector employees.

ACCREDITING ORGANIZATIONS*

In the sections to follow, covering the Joint Commission on Accreditation of Hospitals (JCAH), the American Osteopathic Association (AOA), and the College of American Pathologists (CAP), it should be understood that safety for the medical technologist is but a small and often indirect portion of the accrediting and standard-setting process. However, conditions that are unsafe for the laboratory professional may cause accreditation or licensure to be lost. Laboratory safety is thus directly linked to these processes.

Joint Commission on Accreditation of Hospitals (JCAH)

The JCAH is a *voluntary*, nongovernmental organization. The introduction to the JCAH *Accreditation Manual for Hospitals 1980* states that JCAH seeks to do the following:

1. Establish standards for the operation of hospitals and other health related facilities and services;
2. Conduct survey and accreditation programs that will encourage

*See also Appendix B.

members of the health professions, hospitals and other health related facilities and services voluntarily:

a. To promote high quality care in all aspects in order to give patients the optimal benefits that medical science has to offer,

b. To apply certain basic principles of physical plant safety and maintenance, and of organization and administration of function for efficient care of the patient, and

c. To maintain the essential services in the facilities through coordinated effort of the organized staffs and governing bodies of the facilities;

3. Recognize compliance with standards by issuance of certificates of accreditation;

4. Conduct programs of education and research, and publish the results thereof, which will further the other purposes of the corporation, and to accept grants, gifts, bequests, and devices in support of the purposes of the corporation; and

5. Assure such other responsibilities and conduct such other activities as are compatible with the operation of such standard setting, survey and accreditation programs.

In 1965, Amendment to the Social Security Act, Public Law 89-97, which includes Medicare, was enacted. This law referred to the JCAH and recognized the ability of the health-care sector to voluntarily assess its own participating hospitals. Under the law, JCAH-accredited hospitals were "deemed" to be in compliance with Medicare standards and, therefore, eligible for participation and financial reimbursement. The 1972 Amendment to the Social Security Act, Public Law 92-603, provides for "validation" surveys of these JCAH-accredited hospitals to avoid completely relinquishing control to a nongovernment body.

All JCAH standards are considered by peers as valid, optimal, and achievable, and compliance with them is measurable (see Appendix B). They are also subject to continuous review and revision by specialty and health-care professionals, organizations, experts, and related groups in applicable areas (*e.g.*, National Fire Protection Association, relevant federal agencies, and JCAH surveyors). The standards are comprehensive and applicable to all hospitals that may properly seek accreditation. In seeking to establish substantial overall compliance with JCAH rules, a hospital may, with permission, substitute alternative innovative procedures that provide the desired results. The JCAH accreditation process covers the entire hospital but does have a specific laboratory section as well. The safety standards for the laboratory are found in some of the general hospital safety requirements in addition to those detailed in the laboratory portion. In meeting JCAH standards for accreditation or in complying with Medicare regulations, the hospital laboratory is indirectly assured to be a safer workplace.

American Osteopathic Association (AOA)

The AOA is a voluntary, private organization for osteopathic hospitals that sets standards for accreditation similar to JCAH standards for hospitals.

The AOA standards, *Requirements and Interpretive Guide for Accredited Hospitals of the American Osteopathic Association,* will not be discussed further in this book other than to note that the safety requirements are identical to JCAH standards. These standards may be obtained from the American Osteopathic Association, 212 East Ohio Street, Chicago, IL 60611.

College of American Pathologists (CAP)

The CAP is a national medical specialty organization of more than 9000 board-certified pathologists. It offers, among other services, a laboratory Inspection and Accreditation (I and A) Program that defines standards for laboratory services and their application to individual laboratories. It thus incorporates a continuous form of laboratory inspection by pathologists. The CAP program provides on-site inspections every two years, with self-evaluations in alternate years. The CAP differs from JCAH in its concentration on pathology services alone rather than on the entire hospital. Both are similar, however, in their approach to laboratory safety, which is viewed as a requisite to a well-run laboratory. Providing fast, accurate, and consistently reliable results to the clinician can only be accomplished in a safe and healthful workplace (see Appendix B).

Equivalence

In 1967, the CAP and I and A program earned "equivalent status" with the CDC in the accreditation of interstate laboratories under the Clinical Laboratories Improvement Act of 1967. This enables a hospital to be accredited by either CDC or CAP. In addition, hospitals accredited by the JCAH may now choose the laboratory-inspection portion through CAP rather than JCAH. This avoids duplicate, costly, and time-consuming inspections.

The Health Care Financing Administration (HCFA), which runs the Medicaid and Medicare programs, accepts JCAH accreditation as assurance of compliance with its own regulations. JCAH, in turn, now grants reciprocity to CAP standards. In effect, then, when JCAH certifies a laboratory based on CAP certification, the HCFA considers the HCFA standards met.

OTHER FEDERAL LEGISLATION AFFECTING CLINICAL LABORATORIES

Licensure and inspection of laboratories based on the three federal laws that follow are designed to assure the quality of service to patients (as a prerequisite to government reimbursement) and are not designed to assure safety of laboratory personnel. Four minimum quality-assurance requirements are addressed in these laws. They are the following:

1. Employment of qualified personnel having prescribed prerequisites
2. Development and adherence to an internal quality-control progam
3. Participation in an approved proficiency-testing program
4. Maintenance of facilities, equipment, and records in a manner that assures the accuracy of testing procedures

Clinical Laboratory Improvement Act of 1967 (CLIA 67)

The Clinical Laboratory Improvement Act of 1967 (CLIA 1967) and the rules and regulations set forth under it, apply to laboratories accepting any specimens in interstate commerce and to all laboratories within the District of Columbia. It originally required that these laboratories be licensed to operate by the Communicable Disease Center in Atlanta, Georgia (now called Centers for Disease Control). An exception was made for equivalence if the laboratory was already accredited by the College of American Pathologists (CAP). After some years of differences, CAP and CLIA standards are now essentially identical.

The objective of CLIA 1967 was the assurance of high-quality laboratory services. It was only in pursuit of this goal that a safe and healthful working environment was addressed.

A Public Health Service (PHS)/HCFA Interagency Agreement of 1979 deemed HCFA the sole responsible agency for licensure and inspection under CLIA. HCFA has always been the responsible administrator for the Medicare/Medicaid programs under the Social Security Act.

Medicare—PL 89-97 (Title XVIII of the Social Security Act)

Under Title XVIII of the Social Security Act, HCFA is authorized to license and inspect participating hospitals, including laboratories, as a prerequisite to reimbursement for Medicare payments by the federal government. This law also deemed JCAH accreditation as an acceptable equivalent to HCFA licensure. Any such JCAH-accredited hospital would, therefore, not need an HCFA license or inspection. An amendment in 1972, P.L. 92-603, provided for HCFA to undertake validation surveys of JCAH-accredited hospitals. It should be noted that because JCAH, as of 1979, has accepted CAP inspection and accreditation of laboratories in lieu of its own, CAP may in practice also be an equivalent accreditation substitute for HCFA licensure of Medicare and Medicaid hospital laboratories. As a formality, JCAH accepts responsibility for the CAP accreditation of a laboratory and does not relinquish its equivalence under the law. This situation may be referred to as "subdeeming." The net effect is that one HCFA, JCAH, or CAP inspection will suffice for accreditation and Medicare or Medicaid licensure for the laboratory.

This deemed equivalence serves to save time and money for both hospitals and the Government, and removes unnecessary duplication of inspections and administrative functions.

Medicaid—PL 89-97 (Title XIX of the Social Security Act)

Under Title XIX of the Social Security Act (Section Part A— Hospital Laboratories), the HCFA is authorized to administer Medicaid, a federal/state cooperative program. HCFA sets minimal laboratory quality standards which must be met for federal reimbursement of Medicaid for laboratory services. The states can add to these federal standards but may not weaken them. Each participating hospital must have a state license, although in some states the federal regulations alone satisfy the state. Participation also requires that all applicable state laws and regulations be met and that the hospital itself comply with, and be federally certified under, the Medicare conditions of participation or their equivalent (*e.g.,* JCAH accreditation). In addition to an HCFA or JCAH inspection, state inspections for licensure will also take place. Periodically there is an attempt to consolidate Medicare and Medicaid survey and certification requirements to eliminate differences in interpretation between the two. This approach has not yet been implemented.

Federal requirements for hospitals seeking reimbursement under Medicare or Medicaid extend to the whole hospital. Some states, however, require state approval for only certain procedures (*e.g.,* premarital serology, syphilis serology, phenylketonuria [PKU] testing), and others may review the laboratory by department or as a whole.

Health Care Financing Administration (HCFA) of the Department of Health and Human Services (DHHS)

The HCFA in the Department of Health and Human Services (DHHS) oversees both the Medicare and Medicaid programs and related medical-care quality control. The Medicare program provides basic health benefits to recipients of Social Security and is funded through the Social Security Trust Fund. The Medicaid program, through grants to states, provides medical services to the needy. Before reimbursement is allowed for services provided, HCFA must assure itself, or be assured through reciprocity, of the quality of the health-care service provided. HCFA also develops and monitors health and safety standards for providers of health-care services. It is through these mechanisms that HCFA has a direct relationship with hospital laboratory services and thus indirectly requires safe working conditions for laboratorians. For 13,000 clinical laboratories, HCFA is the federal government's primary regulator. The equivalency status granted to CAP, and now indirectly to JCAH, provides alternate mechanisms for HCFA approval, allowing one inspection per year to satisfy the regulations. Most hospital laboratories come under HCFA rules and regulations because recipients of Medicare and Medicaid are widespread. HCFA affects the day-to-day laboratory more than does any other of the federal agencies.

A primary HCFA goal is the achievement of uniformity in federal laboratory requirements, and HCFA is now well on the road toward achieving this goal. Previously, HCFA had been primarily concerned with maintaining minimum laboratory standards, and CDC and its scientists had focused on how to provide the best possible laboratory services. These philosophical differences are being worked out under the newly transferred responsibilities of the HCFA/CDC Interagency Agreement, giving HCFA licensure authority for those laboratories under CLIA 1967 formerly inspected by CDC. HCFA inspections, therefore, are generally of nonaccredited hospitals and, as far as safety is concerned, use state and local codes as a guide and inspect for obvious hazards to the laboratory worker.

The Centers for Disease Control (CDC)

The CDC has a variety of responsibilities including consultation and assistance in upgrading the performance of clinical laboratories and evaluation and licensing of clinical laboratories engaged in interstate commerce. CDC also develops occupational safety and health standards and performs research through NIOSH, which is a CDC agency.

Laboratories engaged in interstate commerce and laboratories operating in the District of Columbia were formerly licensed and inspected by the CDC. This responsibility has now been transferred to the HCFA as a result of an interagency agreement in 1979 (see preceding section on CLIA 67 under Federal Legislation). It is estimated that millions of federal dollars will be saved annually by consolidation of these responsibilities.

CDC maintains responsibility for developing technical and scientific criteria for occupational standards, developing and administering competency examinations of clinical laboratory personnel, monitoring the effectiveness of state and other third-party evaluation programs, training HCFA inspectors, helping deficient laboratories improve, and researching more efficient evaluation methods. In carrying out these responsibilities, CDC will perform 500 to 1000 follow-up visits per year to already inspected laboratories.

Nuclear Regulatory Commission (NRC)

The Nuclear Regulatory Commission (NRC) is an independent government agency. To protect public and occupational health and safety, as well as the environment, this commission licenses and regulates the uses of nuclear power plants, reactors, reactor fuel, and reactor products including radioisotopes. Licenses are granted both to persons and to companies that own and use radioactive materials. The NRC also inspects the activities of the licensees to ensure that safety rules are not violated.

NRC's responsibilities for ownership and use of radioactive materials bears relevance to hospital laboratory safety. Nuclear-medicine laboratories, because of the relatively high level of radioactive materials used in them, are *strictly* regulated by the NRC. Clinical laboratories, however, doing no more than radioimmunoassay (RIA) or blood culturing with isotope methods, such as the BACTEC system, come under a less strict, broad NRC provision called a *general license* (Fig. 1-4). This general license serves as an exemption from the very strict possession, use, and disposal regulations that would otherwise apply when using high-level radioisotopes. The very low levels of radioactivity in the *in vitro* diagnostic procedures pose little or no threat to the medical technician performing the test. In fact, under the general license it is premissible to discard RIA waste along with the nonradioactive trash after radioactivity labels are removed.

The general license may be issued to any physician, clinical laboratory, or hospital to acquire, possess, or use nuclear by-product materials in pre-packaged form for *in vitro* tests. The strict procedures that must be followed while performing RIA are due to licensure or accreditation regulations, not to the NRC regulations.

Food and Drug Administration (FDA) of the DHHS

The Food and Drug Administration (FDA) is charged with protecting the health of the nation against impure and unsafe foods, drugs, cosmetics, medical devices, and so on. Under an interim organizational realignment, two Centers at the FDA are of relevance to the safety and health of the clinical laboratory worker—these are the National Center for Devices and Radiological Health (NCDRH) and the National Center for Drugs and Biologics (NCDB). Although

NRC Form 483
1-76
10 CFR 31

U.S. NUCLEAR REGULATORY COMMISSION

REGISTRATION CERTIFICATE—IN VITRO TESTING
WITH BYPRODUCT MATERIAL UNDER GENERAL LICENSE

Approved by GAO
38-R0160

Section 31.11 of 10 CFR 31 establishes a general license authorizing physicians, clinical laboratories, and hospitals to possess certain small quantities of byproduct material for *in vitro* clinical or laboratory tests not involving the internal or external administration of the byproduct material or the radiation therefrom to human beings or animals. Possession of byproduct material under 10 CFR 31.11 is not authorized until the physician, clinical laboratory, or hospital has filed NRC Form 483 and received from the Commission a validated copy of NRC Form 483 with registration number.

3. I hereby apply for a registration number pursuant to §31.11, 10 CFR 31 for use of byproduct materials for *(please check one block only)*
☐ a. Myself, a duly licensed physician authorized to dispense drugs in the practice of medicine.
☐ b. The above-named clinical laboratory.
☐ c. The above-named hospital.
4. To be completed by the Nuclear Regulatory Commission.

INSTRUCTIONS
1. Submit this form in triplicate to:
Office of Nuclear Material Safety and Safeguards
ATTN: Radioisotopes Licensing Branch
U.S. Nuclear Regulatory Commission
Washington, D.C. 20555

2. Please print or type the name and address (including zip code) of the registrant physician, clinical laboratory, or hospital for whom or for which this registration is filed. Position the first letter of the address below the left dot and do not extend the address beyond the right dot. (At NRC, a registration number will be assigned and a validated copy of NRC Form 483 will be returned.)

Registration number:

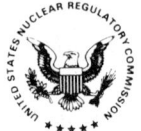

(If this is an initial registration, leave this space blank — number to be assigned by NRC. If this is a change of information from a previously registered general licensee, include your registration number.)

5. If place of use is different from address in Item 1, please give complete address:

6. Certification:

I hereby certify that:

a. All information in this registration certificate is true and complete.

b. The registrant has appropriate radiation measuring instruments to carry out the tests for which byproduct material will be used under the general license of 10 CFR 31.11. The tests will be performed only by personnel competent in the use of the instruments and in the handling of the byproduct materials.

c. I understand that Commission regulations require that any change in the information furnished by a registrant on this registration certificate be reported to the Director of Nuclear Material Safety and Safeguards within 30 days from the effective date of such change.

d. I have read and understand the provisions of Section 31.11 of NRC regulations 10 CFR 31 (reprinted on the reverse side of this form); and I understand that the registrant is required to comply with those provisions as to all byproduct material which he receives, acquires, possesses, uses, or transfers under the general license for which this Registration Certificate is filed with the Nuclear Regulatory Commission.

Date _____   By _____
Signature of person filing form

Printed name and title or position of person filing form

WARNING—18 U.S.C., Section 1001; Act of June 25, 1948; 62 Stat. 749; makes it a criminal offense to make a willfully false statement or representation to any department or agency of the United States as to any matter within its jurisdiction.

Fig. 1-4. NRC registration certificate for *in vitro* testing with byproduct material under general license.

laboratory safety is not the mission of either of these Centers, their efforts do result in improved laboratory safety.

While carrying out programs designed to reduce exposure to ionizing and nonionizing radiation, The Office of Radiological Health (ORH) of the NCDRH has considerable impact on the practice of nuclear medicine. ORH responsibility includes standards development for equipment certification and radiation-control methodology programs. Although not concerned with RIA, the ORH does regulate radiation-emitting equipment (diagnostic and therapeutic), light-scattering systems, and electronic product-radiation emitters.

The Office of Medical Devices (OMD) of the NCDRH develops FDA policy on safety, efficacy, and labeling of medical devices, classifies medical devices, and participates in surveillance and compliance programs for medical devices. The medical devices that are found in the laboratory include all laboratory instruments and *in vitro* diagnostic agents and reagents intended for use in the cure, mitigation, treatment, prevention, or diagnosis of diseases. Obviously, that includes everything from centrifuges and cell counters to pregnancy-testing kits. Although OMD primarily determines the efficacy of the instrument or testing kit, its contents-labeling requirements and performance standards do serve to protect the laboratorian. These labels are a source of vital information to technicians who are working with a multitude of reagents that often are known only by a trade name and may contain ingredients that are hazardous.

The NCDB regulates biological products shipped in interstate and foreign commerce, tests and establishes standards for biologicals, and approves, licenses, and conducts research on new and established biologicals. Such diverse products as *in vivo* skin-test antigens, blood, fractionated blood products, vaccines, hepatitis-test kits, and red-cell typing sera are scrutinized by the NCDB. The NCDB seeks to assure that diagnostic-test kits and *in vivo* products perform as promised, and that *in vivo* products, in addition, be proven safe to administer.

Department of Transportation (DOT)

The Department of Transportation (DOT) has the responsibility to assure national transportation policies and programs conducive to the provision of fast, safe, efficient, and convenient transportation for all modes of travel in the United States. Hazardous materials that traverse the United States, therefore, are regulated by the DOT, which mandates warning labels (Fig. 1-5), hazardous-contents identification, special sturdy or protective packaging, and safe-handling requirements. As far as the laboratory professional is concerned, the DOT thus provides assurance that materials, including biohazards, radioactive products, or hazardous substances, will be visibly labeled and packaged in a manner that will not endanger the person opening the container either in the laboratory or in the receiving room. DOT labeling rules are very strict and apply to potentially hazardous products being shipped interstate no matter how small the size.

Assistant Secretary for Health of the DHHS

The Office of the Assistant Secretary for Health, which reports to and advises the Secretary of Health and Human Services on health-care matters, oversees the PHS agencies, including the CDC, FDA, National Institutes of Health (NIH), and others. The importance of this office to the clinical laboratory lies in laboratory-related recommendations and policies on health care, biomedical research, *and* health-care professionals set forth by the Assistant Secretary for Health. This includes, but is not limited to, allied-health training grants, federal reimbursements for laboratory services, and laboratory inspections. These policy decisions have widespread impact on the performance of laboratory medicine and thus directly affect the operation of all clinical laboratories.

National Institutes of Health (NIH) of the DHHS

The broad mission of the National Institutes of Health (NIH) is to improve the health of the nation. To fulfill this mandate, the NIH conducts and supports biomedical research into the causes, prevention, and cures of diseases, supports research training and the development of research resources, and makes use of modern methods to communicate biomedical information.

NIH is a research and not a regulatory organization; therefore, recommendations for safe working practice in the laboratory made by groups of renowned NIH scientists and science-policy makers are often no more than rules by which their own intra- and extramural researchers must work. Due to the prestige of NIH, however, and to the widespread biomedical funding under their auspices, these recommended safe working procedures are often adopted voluntarily by most other laboratories as a sensible course of action. The NIH guidelines that bear most relevance to the clinical laboratory are those concerning protection against biohazards and carcinogens in the workplace.

Environmental Protection Agency (EPA)

The Environmental Protection Agency (EPA), an independent government agency, was created to protect and enhance our environment to the fullest possible extent under the law. In carrying out this mandate, EPA has direct responsibility for the safe disposal of chemical waste, be it discharged into sewers, released into the atmosphere, or put into landfill sites. Under the Resource Conservation and Recovery Act of 1976 (RCRA), EPA has established regulations to control hazardous-waste disposal. By definition, hazardous-waste disposal includes disposal of liquids if they are reactive, corrosive, toxic, ignitable, or biohazardous. Generally, liquid and solid hospital laboratory wastes are treated or neutralized before they are discharged into sewers, incinerated, or decontaminated and physically carted away. As RCRA regulations now stand, hazardous wastes from hospitals are too small in quantity (<1000 kg per month) for the hospitals to require issuance of EPA RCRA permits as "waste generators." At present, EPA is reevaluating hazardous waste policy and this small-generator exemption will likely undergo change. If more stringent hazardous-waste rules are adopted, this could have a far greater impact on laboratories than it does at present.

Consumer Product Safety Commission (CPSC)

The Consumer Product Safety Commission (CPSC), an independent government agency, serves to protect the public against injury from consumer products, to assist consumers in evaluation of product safety, to develop product-safety standards, and to investigate problems

(Text continues on p. 32)

[30]

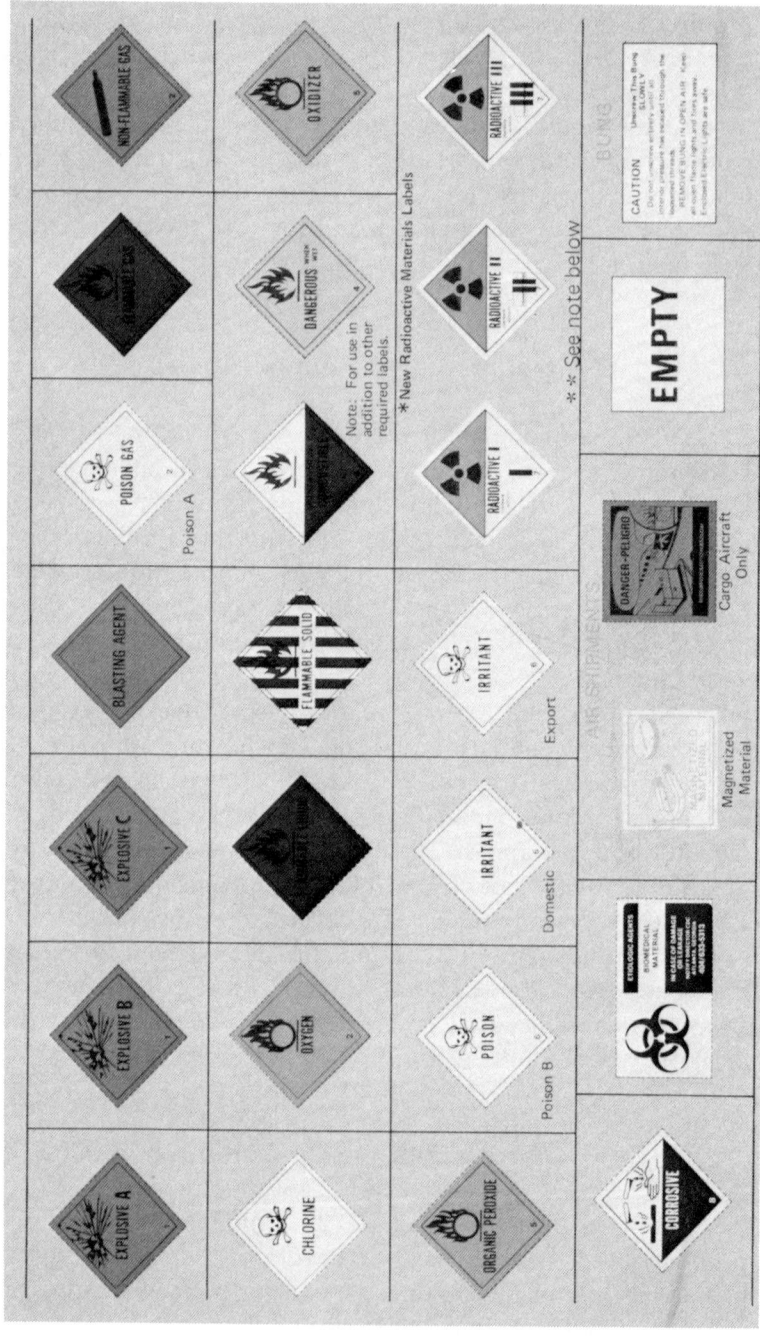

General Guidelines on Use of Labels

1 Each person who offers a hazardous material for shipment must label the package containing the material, if required, with the appropriate label(s). (Sec. 172.400 (a))

2 Labels may be affixed to packages even though not required by the regulations provided each label represents a hazard of the material in the package. (Sec. 172.401)

3 Exceptions to the labeling requirements for limited quantities of certain hazardous materials are specified in the regulations.

4 The number appearing at the bottom corner of some labels represent the UN and IMCO hazard class number. These are permitted, but not required, by DOT regulations. (Sec. 172.407 (g))

5 Label(s), when required, must be affixed to or printed on the surface of the package near the marked proper shipping name. (Sec. 172.406 (a))

6 When two or more different warning labels are required, they must be displayed next to each other. (Sec.172.406 (c))

7 When two or more packages containing compatible hazardous materials are packaged within the same overpack, the outside container must be labeled as required for each class of material contained therein. (Sec. 172.404 (b))

8 Packages containing a sample of a hazardous material other than an explosive must be labeled in accordance with the requirements of Sec. 172.402 (h). (For Explosives, see Title 49, CFR, Part 173, Subpart C)

9 A material classed as an Explosive A, Poison A, or Radioactive material, that also meets the definition of another hazard class, must be labeled as required for each class. (Sec. 172.402 (a))

10 Packages containing Radioactive material, that also meets the definition of one or more additional hazards, must be labeled as a Radioactive material and for each additional hazard on opposite sides of the package. (Sec. 172.403 (e) and (f))

11 A material classed as an Oxidizer, Flammable solid, or Flammable liquid, that also meets the definition of a Poison B, must be labeled POISON, in addition to the hazard class label. (Sec. 172.402 (a) (3))

12 A material classed as a Flammable solid, that also meets the definition of a water reactive material, must have both FLAMMABLE SOLID and DANGEROUS WHEN WET labels affixed. (Sec. 172.402 (a) (4))

NOTE: Printing Errors

RADIOACTIVE MATERIALS LABELS

1. Top portion of RADIOACTIVE I label should be white
2. Red bars on all labels should follow the word RADIOACTIVE

＊
＊

13 For OXYGEN, the word "OXYGEN" may be used in place of the word "OXIDIZER" on the OXIDIZER label. (Sec. 172.405 (a)) For foreign shipments, the NON-FLAMMABLE GAS label may also be required.

14 For CHLORINE, a CHLORINE label may also be used in place of the NON-FLAMMABLE GAS and POISON labels. (Sec. 172.405 (b)) For foreign shipments, the NON-FLAMMABLE GAS label may also be required.

* New labels may be used in lieu of old labels. After January 1, 1982, new labels must be used.

These guidelines do not include all of the DOT hazardous materials labeling and placarding requirements. For details, refer to Title 49, Code of Federal Regulations, Part 172.

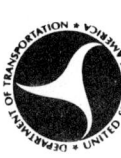

U. S. DEPARTMENT OF TRANSPORTATION
RESEARCH AND SPECIAL PROGRAMS ADMINISTRATION
MATERIALS TRANSPORTATION BUREAU
WASHINGTON, D.C. 20590

Chart 6
FEB 1980

[31]

Fig. 1-5. DOT hazardous materials warning labels.

resulting from consumer use. When a laboratory uses commercial blenders, refrigerators, hot plates, or other such equipment generally purchased from a consumer source, CPSC is the agency responsible for assuring the safety of the product and investigating or removing from the marketplace those items found later to be unsafe. The laboratory is affected by the CPSC in the same manner as is any consumer.

Congressional Committees With Jurisdiction Over Clinical Laboratories

No discussion of regulations and legislation affecting the clinical laboratory can be complete without some mention of the congressional committees that have jurisdiction over them. Whether this jurisdiction is lawmaking or providing funding, the impact can be significant. These are the committees of concern if one is interested in changes in the federal laws affecting the laboratory. These committees are also the points of contact for making one's views known to the lawmakers on current or proposed laboratory-related legislation.

Senate

- Labor and Human Resources Committee (no subcommittee)
- Finance Committee (Health Subcommittee)
- Appropriation Committee (Subcommittee on Labor, Health and Human Services)

House of Representatives

- Energy and Commerce Committee (Health and the Environment Subcommittee)
- Ways and Means Committee (Subcommittee on Health)
- Appropriation Committee (Subcommittee on Labor, Health and Human Services)

The proper address for such correspondence is
  Chairman, (Name of Committee or Subcommittee)
  U.S. Senate
  Washington, DC 20510

or

Chairman, (Name of Committee or Subcommittee)
U.S. House of Representatives
Washington, DC 20515

Others in Brief

Professional Nongovernmental Standard-Setting Organizations

Professional nongovernmental standard-setting organizations such as the Underwriters Laboratories (UL) and the National Fire Protection Association directly affect laboratory safety. UL or a similar organization's approval is necessary on electrical equipment to assure its electrical safety in the clinical laboratory. The relevant National Fire Protection Association Standards (*e.g.,* 101 Life Safety Code and 56C Laboratories in Health Related Institutions) must be met by both new and older health-care institutions when so required by the accreditation procedure or hospital insurance coverage. These codes are often adopted verbatim for state and local fire codes as well.

Professional Organizations

Professional organizations such as the American Society for Medical Technology (ASMT), American Society for Clinical Pathologists (ASCP), and the many varied specialty associations (*e.g.,* American Society for Microbiology) do not write standards or set regulations for laboratory safety but often, through lobbying and raising public and member awareness, are very effective contributors to lawmaking and regulation writing. They also serve to make members conscious of laboratory safety through journals, courses, and guidelines.

State and Local Governments

State and local governmental or regulatory bodies (*e.g.,* health, occupational safety, environmental protection, labor, and fire departments) are not discussed here other than as a reminder that on the state and municipal levels there are often additional layers of governmental organizations and regulations that must be addressed by the hospital.

These sometimes mirror their federal counterparts, but often may be more strict and usually have their own inspection and licensing procedures. Interactions on the state and local levels are often more frequent and more intimately related to the day-to-day functions of the hospital than those at the federal level.

2
Responsibility for Safety and Health

Occupational safety in the clinical laboratory is the result of careful planning, enforcement of a reasonable set of rules, availability of protective equipment, and the use of safety-tested and appropriate instrumentation.

Although subsequent chapters discuss hazardous agents or conditions that pertain especially to one laboratory or another, this chapter covers some roles and responsibilities that pertain to the entire laboratory.

Hospital and laboratory management, laboratory staff, and the employee health service are discussed in relation to maintaining employee safety and health. Although this chapter and the material in subsequent chapters are presented as preferred operating procedures, it should be recognized that this safety material is, in fact, not optional. In reality it is legally, practically, and economically the *only* way to practice good laboratory science.

Good Laboratory Practices for the Clinical Laboratory

- There shall be *no* smoking, eating, drinking, or application of cosmetics in the working area of the laboratory (Figs. 2-1*A* and 2-1*B*).
- Food shall not be stored in laboratory refrigerators or prepared or consumed in laboratory glassware or utensils.
- Laboratory coats or uniforms or protective aprons shall be worn at all times and preferably left in the laboratory at the end of the day.
- Without exception, mouth pipetting of any substance is *not* allowed in the laboratory.
- Each staff member must learn the safety rules and procedures that apply for each laboratory department.
- Potential hazards and appropriate safety precautions should be evaluated before beginning *any* new task.
- Familiarity with all appropriate emergency and protective equipment and procedures is required of each employee.
- Long untied hair, sandals, contact lenses, loose flowing clothing, neckties, and jewelry present hazards that must be minimized or removed.
- Post warning signs when unusual hazards are present.
- When in doubt about any procedure or condition, *ask* before proceeding.
- Spills *must* be cleaned up immediately.
- Return all materials and equipment not in use to storage.
- Do not leave procedures unattended once they are in operation.
- Do not distract or startle another worker or indulge in practical joking or horseplay. Be serious about work practices at all times.
- Use equipment only for its designed purpose.
- Wash hands well before leaving the laboratory area.
- Tidiness, cleanliness, and good housekeeping are required at all work areas; this includes maintaining unobstructed aisles and exits and proper waste handling.
- Unlabeled materials must not be used.
- Adhere to established waste-disposal procedures.
- Do not take shortcuts or take chances with procedures, materials, or equipment.
- Emergency equipment including fire extinguishers, eye washes,

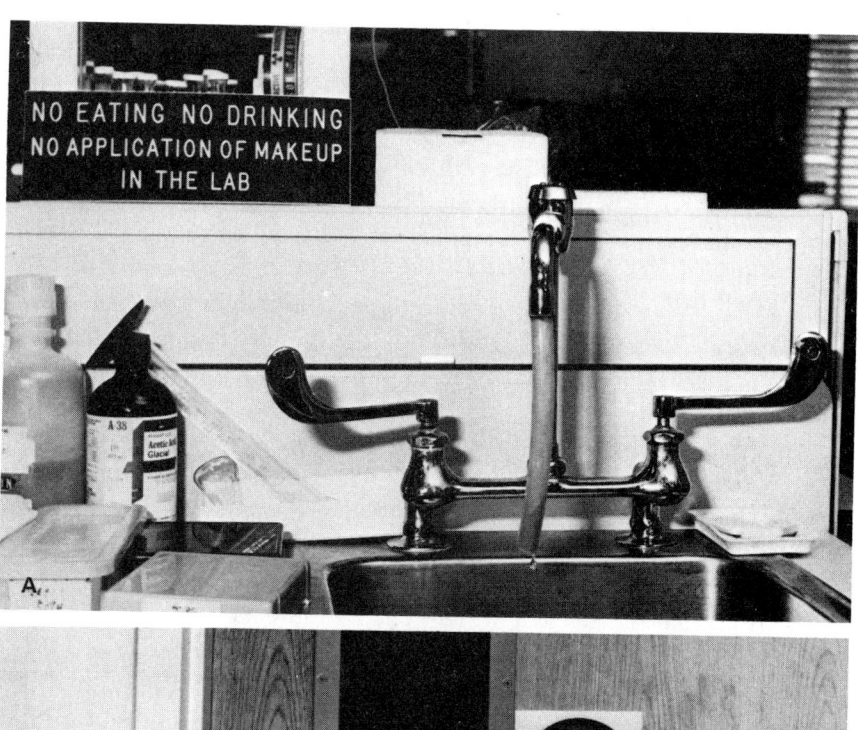

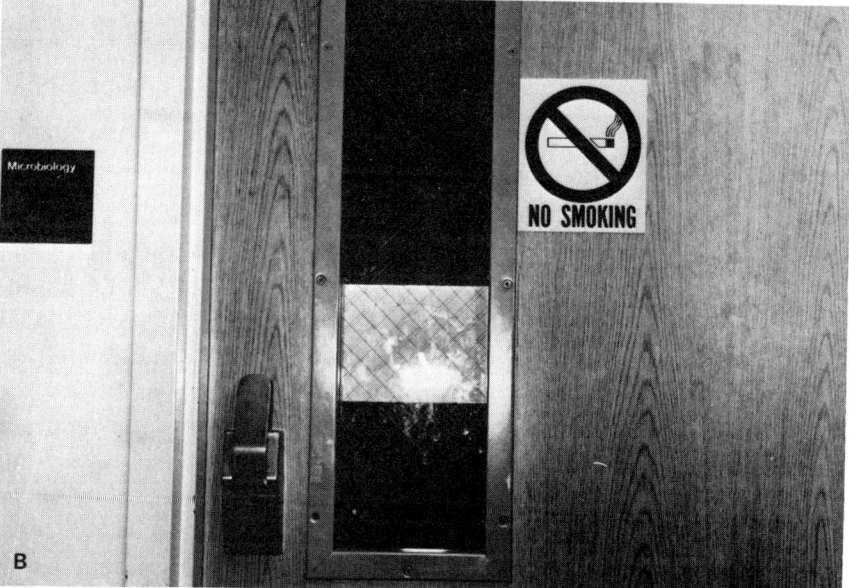

Fig. 2-1*A* **and** *B*. Signs to remind staff of no-smoking, no-eating, and no-drinking rules may be found all over the laboratory. Posted or not, these rules are mandatory. Note the elbow-operated sink in *A*.

and deluge showers shall be routinely inspected and maintained and an inspection record kept.

- All employees shall receive instruction in the use of fire-fighting and protective equipment.
- All equipment shall be routinely inspected and maintained, and an inspection record kept. Needed repairs shall be made immediately or the equipment removed from service until it is repaired.
- All government, accrediting agency, fire-code, and insurance safety rules and regulations for the clinical laboratory shall be enforced. ("Adequate space, facilities, equipment and supplies to perform the services offered with optimum accuracy, precision, efficiency and safety"—see Appendix B.)
- Check laboratory voltage daily with a voltage monitor.
- All employees should know where the main gas and electrical shut-off valves to the entire laboratory are located and how to operate them.
- Illumination at each work bench should be adequate—at least 50 footcandles.

RESPONSIBILITY FOR SAFETY

The Safety Manual

Each laboratory should prepare a laboratory safety manual, which should be readily available to all employees. The safety manual should be tailored to the particular set of circumstances in each clinical laboratory and include the names, phone numbers, and responsibilities of relevant authorized persons including the safety officer, pathologist, laboratory supervisor, laboratory department heads, radiation safety officer, and head of security. It should specify an evacuation plan and provide vital safety and first-aid information. Incident- or accident-reporting procedures, employee health requirements, and emergency plans must also be included, as should well-articulated statements on safety policy and established responsibilities and duties of the safety committee and safety officer.

The ultimate responsibility for day-to-day safety, safe work performance, and knowledge of stated laboratory requirements lies with each employee. The supervisor and chief technologist, however, also bear responsibility for eliminating unsafe practices and conditions in their laboratory when they do occur. Overall laboratory safety responsibility is shared by the staff with the safety officer, who should be authorized to correct and report safety hazards wherever he sees them. The person bearing final responsibility for the safety of *all* laboratory employees is the chief pathologist. To make the system work as it should, the pathologist must rely on and provide support to the safety officer and safety committee and must follow their safety recommendations. Although the pathologist cannot know every violation or breach of good conduct, he can appoint and authorize his staff to make the situation as safe and as compliant with legal guidelines as possible.

Management

Although safety responsibilities of the laboratory staff are the primary topic of this section, a general statement of management's responsibility is an appropriate place to begin.

The safety responsibilities of laboratory management include the following:

- Establishing safety policy
- Providing a safe workplace (including noise, lighting, and temperature considerations)
- Complying with established safety and health standards
- Assessing progress of the safety program
- Reviewing and acting on reports of the following:
     Safety committee
     Safety officer
     Accidents
     Inspection
- Providing facilities (including ventilation, storage space, safety equipment, and monitoring and detection devices) adequate for the task required in the laboratory and requiring that this capacity not be exceeded

To have an effective safety program, then, continuous and dynamic effort and dialogue must occur between "top" and "bottom" elements of the laboratory hierarchy—the management and the staff. Everyone involved in the operation of the laboratory must be safety minded; safety awareness must become a habit, not a chore.

Safety Officer

Each clinical laboratory should have a safety officer with a clearly defined set of duties and responsibilities who answers directly to the pathologist. With the advice and support of the pathologist, the safety officer should develop safety goals, set up and maintain a safety program acceptable to the laboratory and hospital inspection and accrediting agencies, develop and maintain safe working conditions, maintain health records, remedy unsafe conditions, and provide safety education for new and old employees. Although this responsibility appears formidable, the safety officer can and should enlist the help of the safety committee and the laboratory staff in pursuing these objectives.

The safety officer should represent the laboratory in the hospital-wide safety committee and act as liaison between laboratory management and department heads and staff. Because the safety officer is a focal point for safety concerns, he can promote safety awareness, motivate personnel, review and inspect working conditions, uncover problems, and involve all laboratory personnel in safety. The safety officer should attend relevant conferences and training programs and set up a safety library for the staff. At regular intervals, informal safety inspections should be conducted by the safety officer and used as a teaching aid to illustrate safety to the employees. The safety officer should also be responsible for alerting the security staff to what must be monitored when the laboratory is unattended as well as to all other safety-related security matters.

Safety Committee

A laboratory safety committee of perhaps five to ten members is an essential safety component and shares in the work and responsibility of the safety officer. This committee should include representatives of all organizational levels and departments of the laboratory. Members may be appointed or elected and the length of service may vary from one to two years. What is important, however, is that a regular meeting time, perhaps monthly, be set aside during the workday. Minutes should be recorded and an agenda prepared. A major goal of the safety committee is to maintain employee interest in the safety program. Part of each meeting may be devoted to safety education; part should be reserved to review accidents, inspections, and apparent problems. Safety suggestions and questions may be brought up during the review portion of the meeting. Any safety actions taken by laboratory management or by the safety officer should be communicated to the committee at the meeting. Reports from the safety committee should be supplied to the management with written recommendations. The safety officer should chair the safety committee meetings. The problems discussed and the suggestions offered should be transmitted back to the full laboratory staff.

Laboratory Supervisors

The supervisor's responsibility for safety matters in his department is directed toward training employees in general safety techniques as well in as those specific safety matters unique to each procedure. General safety concerns might include wearing an apron, using needle clippers, or chaining a compressed-gas cylinder. Specific safety techniques might include safely attaching a compressed-gas cylinder to an instrument, performing the hepatitis-associated antigen test to minimize aerosols, or transferring a tuberculosis (TB) culture properly in a hood. This careful training is especially critical with new employees to establish an expected level of performance. When the supervisor writes the standard-operating-procedures manual required for the department, safety tips must also be included. The supervisor must also eliminate hazardous conditions or behavior, report on accidents, and make a daily effort to operate the department with a constant awareness of safe working procedures; he also must expect this much effort of each employee.

Laboratory Staff

Employees share in the responsibility for their own safety and the safety of their co-workers. All safety equipment provided must be used as appropriate to the task or situation. Laboratory procedures must be followed without shortcuts or modifications. Injuries, hazards, and accidents must all be reported immediately. Safety education must be an integral part of each job. Good laboratory management will provide and encourage training in safety, whether it is offered on the jobsite or elsewhere. All employees should make every effort to participate on a routine basis whenever safety training is offered. The informal safety audits by the safety officer contribute to alerting the employee to hazards and increase sensitivity to matters of safety in the laboratory. This should be viewed as a positive learning experience, not as punishment. The employee who performs in a safe and aware manner is, of course, not assuring only his own well-being but also that of fellow workers.

RESPONSIBILITY FOR HEALTH

Employee Health Services

The employee health service in the hospital performs myriad functions, among them keeping absenteeism, personnel turnover, and worker's compensation to a minimum. Checking the spread of disease between patients and staff is an additional and vital goal of the employee health service in the hospital setting; this is *not* a concern for the employee health service in a nonhospital setting. The patients and the laboratory work itself do present serious potential insults to the health of the medical technologist.

Clinical-laboratory personnel are exposed to infection and disease through contact with blood, tissues, body fluids, and culture specimens and through direct patient contact. In addition, the daily routine of the laboratory presents added exposure to hazards including flammables, toxic substances, corrosives, radiation, and electricity.

Assuming that the employee adheres to proper work procedures and that the environment is as safe as it reasonably can be, a vigilant employee health service can help the laboratory employees to remain healthy despite the occasional accidents that do occur. Often, practical instruction and helpful suggestions are provided by the employee health unit in such matters as disease prevention, bringing illness or injury promptly to medical attention, and infection-control techniques. The total environment of the worker affects his value and production as an employee. Concern for this through the practice of a rigorous occupational-health program reassures the employee of management interest in his total and work-related well-being.

The employee health service should provide the following:

1. *Physical examinations*
   a. *Preplacement physical examinations* are used to place an employee in work for which he is physically, mentally, and emotionally qualified. The worker should be in a position in which his health is not at risk and in which he does not present a risk to others. Often the preplacement physical is a legal requirement. The preplacement physical should include the following:
      • History and physical examination, weight and height measurements, blood-pressure reading, pulse and respiration rates, temperature reading, audiogram, visual test, urinalysis, determination of hemoglobin and hematocrit, complete blood count, routine chemistry tests, a Pap smear, a serologic test for syphilis, chest x-ray examination or TB skin test, and electrocardiogram (ECG). Assessment of mental and emotional state may be included.
   b. *Samples of employee sera* may be drawn at the time of employment, and often a battery of chemistry tests is run then also. This provides a sample of "baseline" values, which represent the condition of the employee when he started his job. These values can be used to establish the occupational relatedness of a disease or to rule out a suspected illness if a rise in antibody titer over the baseline level cannot be shown.

2. *Periodic health evaluations*
   Periodic health evaluations are performed to ensure that the worker's health has not been unduly affected and that he is able to handle his job, to encourage him in proper health care, and to provide early treatment for minor nondisabling conditions. Every employee working with specific health hazards should be examined periodically and appropriate observations should be made as required by the hazard. For example, workers exposed to severe stress, TB organisms, toxic chemicals, or radiation require different screening and follow-up examinations. Employees with special medical conditions such as pregnancy, diabetes, heart conditions, allergies, and injuries should be

examined periodically to determine their fitness to continue working at a particular task and to evaluate their condition on a continuing basis.

3. *Approval of return from sick leave*

Any employee returning after being away from work for more than 3 days for illness should provide the employee health unit or emergency room with a note from his doctor giving the reason for his absence and his doctor's approval to return to work. The employee health unit or emergency room must also approve the employee's return to work before the employee may resume duties. This is done to be certain that the person is truly able to return to work, to establish whether he is able to return to the same job, to alert the occupational-health personnel to any potential public health problem, and to determine whether the illness might be related to his occupation. It also provides some protection to patients and co-workers.

4. *Treatment of illness and injuries*

The employer is responsible for providing medical diagnosis and treatment of job-related illness and injury. The ill employee should be encouraged to visit the employee health unit, where the job relatedness of his disease may be diagnosed. Often, the health unit may have knowledge of hospitalwide epidemics at their onset or be aware early on of hazardous conditions that may cause problems for more than one employee. The health unit or the laboratory will fill out a report form for each employee injury or illness (Fig. 2-2). Copies are sent to various departments where such information is tallied and retained.

5. *Provision of medical care for other reasons*

The employee health unit also provides medical care for the following:

- Emergency occupational injuries and illnesses
- Nonoccupational conditions—to keep the worker on the job
- Emergency nonoccupational conditions—to protect the employee until he can be placed in the care of his own physician.
- Maintenance of health through education, immunization, infection-control surveys, Pap smears, and counseling

Personnel suffering illness or injury during regular working hours should be sent to the employee health unit. If the health-related problem arises during the evening, night, or weekend

• *MUST BE COMPLETED AND FORWARDED TO EMPLOYEE HEALTH WITHIN 48 HOURS OF INCIDENT.* •

NAME OF INJURED		AGE	SOCIAL SECURITY NO.	EMPL. NO.	DATE/TIME OF INCIDENT	WAS EMPLOYEE ON DUTY?
						☐ YES ☐ NO
ADDRESS (street, city, state, zip)						

DESCRIPTION OF INCIDENT & EXTENT OF INJURY

HOW AND WHERE DID THE INCIDENT OCCUR?

WHAT WAS EMPLOYEE DOING AT THE TIME OF THE INCIDENT?

WHAT WERE THE CONTRIBUTING FACTORS?

ARE THERE ANY PRIOR INJURIES/PRE-EXISTING PHYSICAL CONDITIONS?

EMPLOYEE WAS TREATED:	EMERGENCY RM.	EMPLOYEE HEALTH	DISPOSITION (IF KNOWN)	RETURNED TO DUTY	SENT HOME	OTHER:

SIGNATURE OF EMPLOYEE ▶_____

DATE

REPORT OF SUPERVISOR'S INVESTIGATION

UNSAFE CONDITIONS: DESCRIBE ANY UNSAFE CONDITIONS INVOLVING MACHINERY, EQUIPMENT, BUILDING OR PREMISES, ETC.

UNSAFE ACT: WHAT WAS DONE INCORRECTLY?

ACTION TAKEN: WHAT HAS BEEN DONE TO CORRECT THE CONDITION CAUSING THE INCIDENT?

PREVENTION: WHAT CAN BE DONE TO PREVENT FURTHER INCIDENTS LIKE THIS?

ACCIDENT AREA	DATE	ACCIDENT AREA SUPERVISOR'S SIGNATURE ▶
EMPLOYEE'S DEPT. HEAD SIGNATURE (IF DIFFERENT FROM ACCIDENT AREA) ▶		ACCIDENT AREA DEPT. HEAD'S SIGNATURE ▶

/84 44JXXX   EMPLOYEE HEALTH

Fig. 2-2. Report of employee occupational injury/illness.

shift, the employee should be directed to the emergency room
for treatment. Although the relationship between an employee
and his personal physician must not be interfered with, the
employee health unit can and should routinely provide medical
care for non–job-related conditions such as flu, allergies, rashes,

a need for blood-pressure checks, and so on. The employee should always report any significant change in his health status to the employee health service for his permanent record.

Immunizations and injections required or provided by the employee health unit depend on the type of work of the employee, the disease or illness he has contracted or been exposed to, and the hospital policy. Although the employee health unit might routinely provide flu shots or similar injections to employees and perform injections for allergic patients, policies may vary as to the administration of prophylactic γ-globulin for hepatitis exposures and needle-stick injuries. Other preventive measures for various employee infections or toxic-substance exposures also vary from hospital to hospital.

The employee health unit is expected to produce an annual report, by hospital department, on the number and kind of accidents and illnesses it services each year. OSHA standards also require that records be kept on the monitoring and control of environmental hazards. Most hospital health units treat more puncture wounds than any other kind of injury (see Chap. 5).

The employee health unit should be consulted on decisions regarding job placement of pregnant or reproductive-age women. Although general laboratory work does *not* present a special hazard to these women, certain individual and collective considerations for them must be addressed. Usually the health unit, the employee, and the employee's own physician are all consulted. Considerations for pregnant or reproductive-age women include the following:

- Whether to give vaccines, injections, or x-ray examinations to pregnant or possibly pregnant workers after they are exposed at work to an illness or after they sustain a puncture wound
- To determine the amount and kind of patient contact that is to be allowed and for what term of the pregnancy (*e.g.*, contact between the pregnant worker and the patient in isolation)
- To determine a policy on the extent of work in nuclear medicine that is allowed the pregnant worker (radioimmunoassay is not considered a hazard to the pregnant worker)
- Whether to allow the pregnant employee or possibly preg-

nant employee to perform phlebotomies or hepatitis-antigen testing

Coordination

The health unit should consistently and continuously provide health, safety, and environmental information for all employees and coordinate these services with the laboratory safety officer. This should include information on the use of the health unit, including the reporting of injury and illness. Both men and women in their reproductive years should be advised of any known or potential work-related hazards affecting conception and pregnancy.

Confidential employee medical records kept by the health unit should include the results of physicals, radiation exposures, and other safety and health matters relating to the individual employee.

It should be apparent that the employee health unit operates to its maximum potential when it has effective communication with the various departments, services, unions, and safety and infection-control committees.

3
Clinical Chemistry

The average clinical chemistry laboratory includes an array of electrical instruments, computers, chemicals, centrifuges, glassware, specimens, mixers, and heating devices. The hazards represented by this array include flammables, corrosives, suspected carcinogens, pressurized gases, aerosols, and poisons. A more substantive look at what is actually occurring in the laboratory reveals that dozens of different tests are performed and hundreds, if not thousands, of test results are produced daily. Telephone responses are made continuously to stat inquiries, and stat orders are taken. Specimens are always arriving for one test or another, and supplies are continuously replenished by the laboratory staff.

Safety equipment, fire extinguishers, spill-cleanup kits, fire blankets, emergency eye washes and showers, safety pipettes, and goggles are among the chemicals and instruments. Technicians carefully performing work at their benches follow precautions required by the general laboratory rules and the specific hazards of the chemical procedures in which they are engaged. How does this complicated laboratory, with its diversity of tests and hazards, function so well?

Obviously, good management and planning are essential. Beyond that, the setting of and adherence to strict rules of safety keep the chemistry laboratory functioning smoothly despite the hazards and workload.

This chapter examines the hazards encountered in the chemistry laboratory and discusses the safety procedures and the safety equipment mandatory in this setting. It is evident that the vast test output and the low accident rate in the chemistry laboratory are *not* "accidental," but rather are achieved through hard work and knowledge. The chapter begins with a discussion of hazard classification and some examples of widely accepted classification systems. The major chemical hazards in clinical chemistry are then covered in some detail, with examples of each; these are flammables, combustibles, oxidizers (including peroxide formers), corrosives, and toxic substances. Following this, an approach to the safe use of accessory chemistry equipment (excluding computers and large automated instruments) is presented. The topics of ventilation, storage, chemical labeling; spills, and waste disposal are addressed in the remaining pages of the chapter. Summaries of good laboratory practices for reagent handling and glassware safety are provided for reference at the end of the chapter.

HAZARDS IN THE CLINICAL LABORATORY

Classification of Hazards in the Clinical Laboratory

The National Institute for Occupational Safety and Health (NIOSH) has defined *hazardous materials* as "a substance or mixture of substances having properties capable of producing adverse effects on the health or safety of the worker" and, in addition, are "toxic, flammable or reactive." A NIOSH study of these hazardous workplace materials found thousands of hazardous materials identified only by trade names, many materials unrecognized as hazards, many unrecognized exposures, and total lack of uniformity and completeness in the labeling and identification of hazards. They also found a greater than expected ignorance of hazardous substances by employer and employee alike (*Federal Register,* Vol. 46, No. 11, Jan. 16, 1981).

Satisfactory systems do exist for hazards identification, but there is no requirement that they be used. A discussion of several such systems follows.

All chemicals can be classified and labeled according to the predominant hazard they present (Figs. 3-1 and 3-2). Such classification provides guidance in the handling, storage, use, and disposal of the chemical. Hazard classification is, unfortunately, not a simple matter and several comprehensive classification systems are in use (see examples on page 52).

A standard, universally recognized hazard classification system provides the best assurance of being readily understood everywhere and minimizes dangerous ambiguities. The system that comes closest to this ideal is the United Nations Hazard Classification (Table 3-1). The U.N. system is required by the U.S. Department of Transportation (DOT) on all chemicals transported in the United States and contiguous waters. All chemicals fit into at least one of the U.N. hazard classes, but the

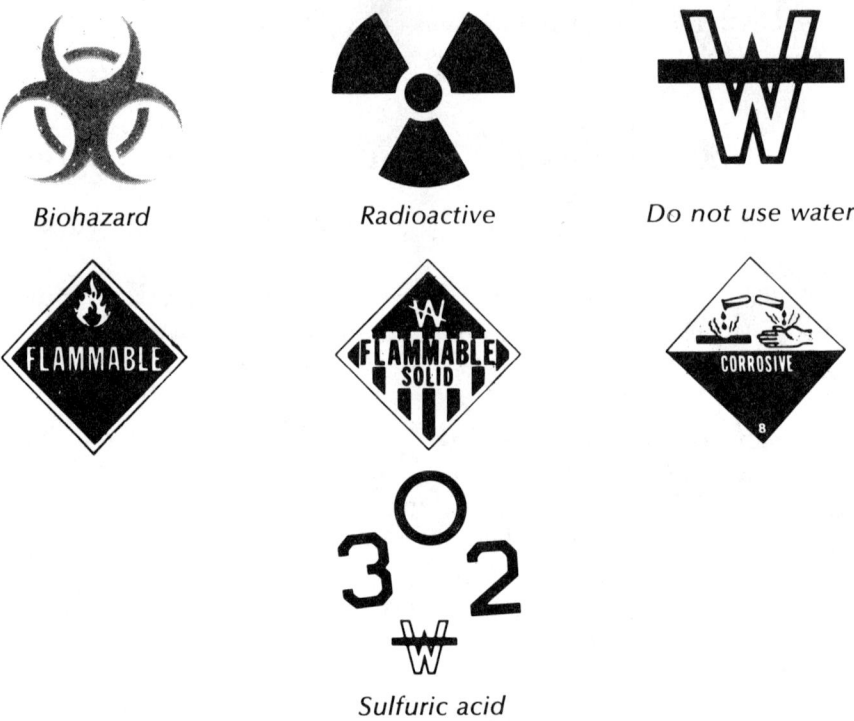

Biohazard   *Radioactive*   *Do not use water*

Sulfuric acid

Fig. 3-1. Hazard symbols.

CAUTION

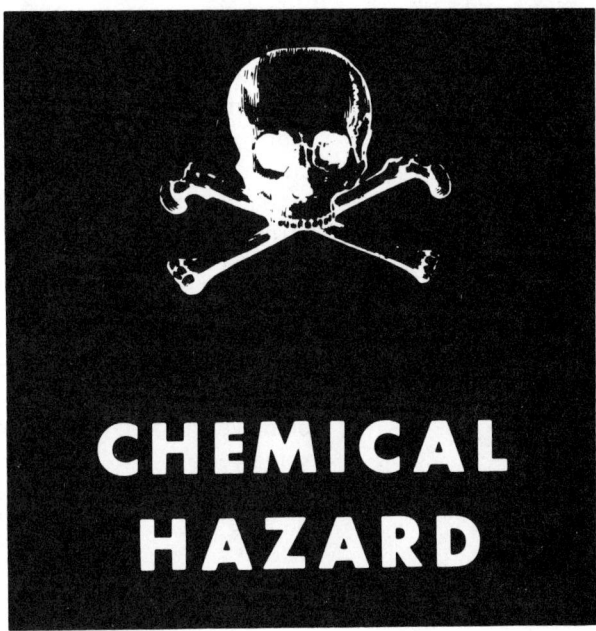

Fig. 3-2. Chemical-hazard warning sign.

process of classification is complicated by the multitude of names given to some chemicals and the fact that many chemicals present several hazards. Additionally, chemicals are often hazardous because of circumstances under which they are used (*e.g.,* with boiling water) rather than because of inherent properties (*e.g.,* as with sulfuric acid). Clinical laboratories deal with all of the nine classes of hazardous materials in the U.N. Hazard Classification and, therefore, laboratory staff must understand the nine hazards and how to work with them. As a comprehensive starting place, essential and useful information on each chemical in the laboratory can and should be obtained from the *Material Safety Data Sheet.* These should be kept on file for all laboratory chemicals and are valuable aids in preventing and minimizing accidents with chemicals (Fig. 3-3).

(Text continues on p. 54)

EXAMPLES OF HAZARD CLASSIFICATION SYSTEMS

National Hazards Control Institute Hazardous Materials Octagon†

- Corrosive
- Radioactive
- Flammable
- Thermal
- Explosive
- Pressure
- Reactive
- Toxic

U.S. Environmental Protection Agency

- Ignitability
- Corrosivity
- Reactivity
- Toxicity
- Radioactivity
- Infectiousness
- Phytotoxicity
- Teratogenicity and mutagenicity

Steere—Safety in the Chemical Laboratory†

- Mechanical
- Electrical
- Ionizing
- Nonionizing
- Biological and micro-biological
- Chemical
- Atmospheric pressure differentials
- Thermal nonfire
- Fire

United Nations* U.S. Department of Transportation

- Explosives
- Compressed gases
- Flammable liquids
- Flammable solids
- Oxidizing materials
- Poisonous materials
- Radioactive materials
- Corrosive materials
- Other

Best's Safety Directory†

- Unstable
- Combustible
- Corrosive
- Explosive
- Oxidizer
- Reactive
- Toxic
- Radioactive

*See Table 3-1.
†See bibliography for publication information.

Table 3-1. Classifying Hazardous Materials

GENERAL CLASSIFICATION U.N./DOT CLASSIFICATIONS	EXAMPLES	HAZARDOUS PROPERTIES

Poisonous materials
  Poison
  Irritant
  Etiologic agent
	Benzene, sulfur dioxide
	Trichloroacetic acid
	Anthrax, botulism, rabies
		Harm from inhalation, ingestion, absorption, effect on environment

Radioactive materials	Iodine^{123}, iodine^{131}, cobalt^{60}, plutonium	Harm—injure living tissues, internal and external
Corrosive materials	Acids—hydrochloric acid, sulfuric acid, nitric acid Bases—caustic soda, caustic potash	Harm—injure living tissues, internal and external; oxidizing effect; splatter potential
Other	Dry ice, carbon tetrachloride Metallic mercury Bleaching powder Disinfectants	Noxious Corrosive
Explosives	Sodium azide, TNT	Sensitive to heat and shock; contamination could cause explosion; thermal and mechanical effects

Compressed gases
  Flammable gas
  Nonflammable gas
 	
Special forms
  Liquefied
 	
  Cryogenic
  Gas in solution
	Acetylene, butane, hydrogen
	Carbon dioxide, nitrogen, sulfur dioxide
	
	Butane, LNG, nitrogen, propane
	
	Ethylene, hydrogen, nitrogen
	Acetylene
		BLEVE (fireball) potential
		Vapor–air explosion potential
		Flammability hazard; highly mobile vapors; toxicity, corrosivity potentials
		Liquefied gases—cold temperatures—frostbite—expansion ratio high

Flammable liquids
  Pyrophoric liquid
  Flammable liquid
  Combustible liquid
	Aluminum alkyls, alkyl
	Boranes, acetone, methyl
	Alcohol
		Flammability
		Explosion potential BLEVE (fireball) Vapor/air
		Potentially corrosive, toxic, thermally unstable

(continued)

Table 3-1. Classifying Hazardous Materials (continued)

GENERAL CLASSIFICATION U.N./DOT CLASSIFICATIONS	EXAMPLES	HAZARDOUS PROPERTIES

Flammable solids
  Water reactive
  Spontaneously
    combustible
	Magnesium
	Calcium carbide, sodium
	hydrides, phosphorus, sodium,
	  potassium
		Readily ignite and burn explo-
		  sively, some spontaneously
		Water reactive potentials yield
		  heat and gas
		Toxic and corrosive potentials

Oxidizing materials
  Oxidizer
  Organic peroxide
	Ammonium nitrite, sodium
	  nitrate, benzoyl peroxide,
	  peracetic acid, chromates,
	  perchlorates, nitrites, bio-
	  mates, chlorites
		Supply oxygen to support com-
		  bustion of normally nonflam-
		  mable materials, yielding heat;
		  explosively sensitive to heat,
		  shock, friction; toxicity
		  potential

Adapted from Wright CJ: Recognition and Control of Hazardous Materials. Fire Technology Program, Western Kentucky University, 1978.

When assessing a potential chemical or procedural hazard, the following factors should be considered and prepared for by the laboratory supervisor and technicians:

- Temperature sensitivity
- Impact sensitivity
- Flammability properties
- Pressure development
- Reactive energy
- Reaction rate
- Effects of volume or mass
- Concentration
- Contamination
- Catalysis
- Peroxide formation
- Effects of air and water
- Compatibility
- Chemical structure

(Text continues on p. 58)

U.S. DEPARTMENT OF LABOR
Occupational Safety and Health Administration

Form Approved
OMB No. 44-R1387

MATERIAL SAFETY DATA SHEET

Required under USDL Safety and Health Regulations for Ship Repairing,
Shipbuilding, and Shipbreaking (29 CFR 1915, 1916, 1917)

SECTION I

MANUFACTURER'S NAME	EMERGENCY TELEPHONE NO.

ADDRESS *(Number, Street, City, State, and ZIP Code)*

CHEMICAL NAME AND SYNONYMS	TRADE NAME AND SYNONYMS

CHEMICAL FAMILY	FORMULA

SECTION II · HAZARDOUS INGREDIENTS

PAINTS, PRESERVATIVES, & SOLVENTS	%	TLV (Units)	ALLOYS AND METALLIC COATINGS	%	TLV (Units)
PIGMENTS			BASE METAL		
CATALYST			ALLOYS		
VEHICLE			METALLIC COATINGS		
SOLVENTS			FILLER METAL PLUS COATING OR CORE FLUX		
ADDITIVES			OTHERS		
OTHERS					

HAZARDOUS MIXTURES OF OTHER LIQUIDS, SOLIDS, OR GASES	%	TLV (Units)

SECTION III · PHYSICAL DATA

BOILING POINT (°F.)		SPECIFIC GRAVITY (H$_2$O=1)	
VAPOR PRESSURE (mm Hg.)		PERCENT, VOLATILE BY VOLUME (%)	
VAPOR DENSITY (AIR=1)		EVAPORATION RATE (_____ =1)	
SOLUBILITY IN WATER			
APPEARANCE AND ODOR			

SECTION IV · FIRE AND EXPLOSION HAZARD DATA

FLASH POINT (Method used)	FLAMMABLE LIMITS	Lel	Uel
EXTINGUISHING MEDIA			
SPECIAL FIRE FIGHTING PROCEDURES			
UNUSUAL FIRE AND EXPLOSION HAZARDS			

PAGE (1)   *(Continued on reverse side)*   Form OSHA-20
Rev. May 72

Fig. 3-3. An example of a material safety data sheet. These should be kept on file for all chemicals used in the laboratory and requested from the manufacturer for chemicals ordered for the first time.

NFPA 704. IDENTIFICATION OF THE HAZARDS OF MATERIALS

NFPA 704. *Identification of the Hazards of Materials* is a symbol system intended for use on fixed installations such as laboratory entrances and storerooms. It provides, at a glance, an indication of the inherent hazards of the chemicals within, as well as the severity of these hazards under *emergency* conditions. The diamond identifies the health, flammability, and reactivity hazards of the chemicals and indicates the severity of each by use of a 0–4 numerical gradient placed in the upper three squares of the diamond. The 0 indicates the lowest degree of hazard; the 4, the highest. The fourth square, at the bottom, is used for special information. This system is designed to be simple, easily understood, interpreted quickly in poor light, and adequate for emergencies at the expense of some specificity and comprehensiveness.

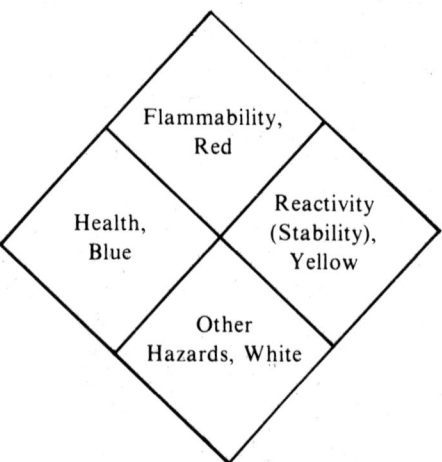

The five degrees of hazard have these meanings to fire fighters:*

4—Too dangerous to approach with standard fire-fighting equipment and procedures. Withdraw and obtain expert advice on how to handle.

3—Fire can be fought using methods intended for extremely hazardous situations, such as unmanned monitors or

*Reproduced from the Fire Protection Handbook, 15th ed. Copyright © 1981, National Fire Protection Association, Quincy, Massachusetts. Reproduced by permission.

personal protective equipment which prevents all bodily contact.

2—Can be fought with standard procedures, but hazards are present which require certain equipment or procedures to handle safely.

1—Nuisance hazards present which require some care, but standard firefighting procedures can be used.

0—No special hazards, therefore, no special measures.

Health Hazards

4—Materials too dangerous to health to expose fire fighters. A few whiffs of the vapor could cause death. Protective clothing and breathing apparatus available to the average fire department will not provide adequate protection against inhalation or skin contact with these materials.

3—Materials extremely hazardous to health but areas may be entered with *extreme* care.

2—Materials hazardous to health but areas may be entered freely with self-contained breathing apparatus.

1—Materials only slightly hazardous to health.

0—Materials which on exposure under fire conditions, should offer no health hazard beyond that of ordinary combustible material.

Flammability Hazards

4—Very flammable gases or very volatile flammable liquids.

3—Materials that can be ignited under almost all normal temperature conditions. Water may be ineffective because of the low flash point of the materials.

2—Materials that must be moderately heated before ignition will occur. Water spray may be used to extinguish the fire because the material can be cooled below its flash point.

1—Materials that must be preheated before ignition can occur. Water may cause frothing if it gets below the surface of the liquid and turns to steam. However, water fog gently applied to the surface will cause a frothing which will extinguish the fire.

0—Materials that will not burn.

(continued)

Reactivity (Stability) Hazards

The rating also identifies the level of reactivity.

4—Materials which are readily capable of detonation at normal temperatures and pressures. If they are involved in a massive fire, vacate the area.

3—Materials which, when heated and under confinement, are capable of detonation and that may react violently with water. Fire fighting should be conducted from behind explosion-resistant locations.

2—Materials which will undergo a violent chemical change at elevated temperatures and pressures but do not detonate.

1—Materials which are normally stable but may become unstable in combination with other materials or at elevated temperatures and pressures. Use normal precautions as in approaching any fire.

0—Materials which are normally stable and, therefore, do not produce any reactivity hazard to fire fighters.

Other Hazards

Adaptations of the NFPA 704 use a variety of symbols in the other-hazards category. Figure 3-1 shows examples of some easily understood symbols. The 704 standard suggests only the radioactive pinwheel and the W (which indicates that water use may cause a hazard) for this square, not the other symbols.

In assessment of a potential hazard, under no circumstances should the following energy sources be overlooked as their impacts on the chemicals or procedures can be devastating:

- Flames
- Sparks
- Hot surfaces
- Friction
- Compression
- Impact
- Vibration
- Light
- Spontaneous combustion
- Rapid pressure changes

As previously stated, all of the hazards found in the U.N. Hazard Classification System are found in the clinical laboratory. For this reason, it is important to provide some background material on each type of hazard and to illustrate the conditions under which each hazard may occur in the laboratory. Corrosives, flammables (including combustibles), explosives, oxidizers (including peroxide formers), and toxics (poisons) will be covered in this chapter. Biohazards, radiation, and compressed gases are covered in other chapters. For the purpose of the clinical laboratory, the safety precautions given for oxidizers and flammables will provide sufficient protection to avoid explosive conditions.

Corrosives

Corrosives are listed in Tables 3-2, 3-3, and 3-4. Corrosives used in the clinical chemistry laboratory can be described as acids or bases that etch flesh with first-, second-, or third-degree burns 24 hours after contact. Some corrosives destroy live tissue as they penetrate it; others cause damage after they have penetrated well into deeper tissues. The former produce pain, itching, skin discoloration, or fumes; the latter, which are far more insidious, migrate into tissues and cause deep, serious burns. The corrosives that cause delayed effects tend to be the most damaging. Inhalation of corrosive vapors or ingestion of corrosives causes severe edema and extensive burning of the respiratory tract or mouth and throat.

Surprise is another dangerous aspect of corrosives. Pain and shock contribute to the panic that disorients the corrosives victim and often cause eye-wash fountains and safety showers to be forgotten. Someone else must force the victim to thoroughly wash the corrosive away. In the case of eye burns, this may include holding the victim's eye open to irrigate the eye properly. When skin is burned with a corrosive, immediate irrigation of the affected skin (or eye) is essential and must continue for a full 15 minutes to prevent or minimize damage. Chemical neutralizers must *not* be applied to the skin.

All containers of corrosive acids and bases should be labeled with both a *CORROSIVE* and a *DANGER* label. To protect the eyes, goggles and other protective equipment should be worn when working with corrosives. Shields or aprons should be used when necessary. Corrosives should *not* be placed above eye level and ideally should sit in a tray or container large enough to confine the contents in case of an accident. A working eye-wash fountain and safety shower are essential in working with corrosives, as is adequate ventilation or a hood to minimize buildup of vapors. A commercial spill kit with chemical neutralizers is the best method for cleanup of a corrosives spill.

Among the corrosives that may be encountered in the laboratory are solids (caustic alkaline hydroxides, sulfides, carbonates, and sodium, potassium, lithium, phosphorus, magnesium, chromium and their salts) and liquids (mineral acids, organic acids, and solutions of strong bases and organic solvents).

Table 3-2. Corrosive Liquids Commonly Used in the Laboratory

CORROSIVE LIQUID	CORROSIVENESS AND TOXICITY*	HAZARD IDENTIFICATION†			
		HEALTH	FLAMMABILITY	REACTIVITY	OTHER
Acids					
Acetic	E, S	2	2	1	
Carbolic (phenol)	Sy, E, S (severe burns)	3	2	0	Lethal
Cresylic (cresol)	Sy, E, S	3	2	0	
Formic	S	3	2	0	
Hydrochloric	Sy, E, S, URT, GI	3	0	0	
Nitric	Sy, E, S, URT, GI	3	0	1	Oxidizer, explosive
Oxalic	Sy, S, GI	2	1	0	
Perchloric	E, S, GI	3	0	3	Oxidizer
Phosphoric	E, S, GI	2	0	0	
Picric	E, S, URT, GI	2	4	4	Oxidizer, explosive
Sulfuric	E, S, GI (deep burns)	3	0	2	W̶
Trichloroacetic	E, S, GI	3	2	1	
Solvents	E, S	1–2	3–4	0	

*Symbols used for corrosive and toxic effects

  Sy = systemic   URT = upper respiratory tract
  E = eyes   GI = gastrointestinal tract
  S = skin

†For explanation of the hazard rating system (0–4), see Hazard Identification System.
Sodeman TM: Clinical laboratory safety. Lab Med 11, No. 8:1980.

Table 3-3. Corrosive Solids Commonly Used in the Laboratory

CORROSIVE SOLID	CORROSIVENESS AND TOXICITY*	HAZARD IDENTIFICATION†			
		HEALTH	FLAMMABILITY	REACTIVITY	OTHER
Alkali metals					
Na, K, Li (and salts)	E, S (deep burns)	3	1	2	W
Alkali earth metals					
Ca, Mg, Ba (and salts)	E, S	1	1	2	W
Transition elements					
I, Fe, Hg (and salts)	SY, S	1–3	2	1	
Compounds					
Disulfides	S	1	0	0	
Carbonates	S	1–2	0	0	
Cyanates	Sy, E, S	3	0	0	Poison
Dichromates	S	1–2	0	1	Oxidizer
Ferricyanates	S	1	0	0	
Hydroxides	E, S, GI	1–3	0	1	
Oxides	E, S, URT	1–2	0	1	
Permanganates	E, S	1–2	0	1	Oxidizer

*Symbols used for corrosive and toxic effects
  Sy = systemic
  E   = eyes
  S   = skin
  URT = upper respiratory tract
  GI   = gastrointestinal tract
†For explanation of the hazard rating system (0–4), see Hazard Identification System.
 Sodeman TM: Clinical laboratory safety. Lab Med 11, No. 8:1980.

Flammables—Theory and Definitions

For the purpose of this section, the definitions and hazards referred to as flammables are the flammable *liquids*—liquids at normal temperature (70°F) and pressure (14.7 psi) although, depending on temperature and pressure conditions, liquids can become solids or gases

Table 3-4. Corrosive Gases Commonly Used in the Laboratory

CORROSIVE GAS	CORROSIVENESS AND TOXICITY*	HAZARD IDENTIFICATION†			
		HEALTH	FLAMMABILITY	REACTIVITY	OTHER
Group I					
Ammonia	Sy, URT	2	1	0	
Acetic acid	Sy, URT	2	2	1	
Carbolic acid (phenol)	Sy, URT	3	2	0	Poison
Formaldehyde	Sy, URT	2	2	0	
Hydrochloric acid	Sy, URT	3	0	0	
Nitric acid	Sy, URT	3	0	0	Oxidizer
Fuming sulfuric acid	Sy, URT	3	0	2	W̶
Group II					
Asphyxiant gases; not direct corrosives	Sy	1–3	2–4	0	Anesthetic
Group III					
Aliphatic hydro-carbons‡	Sy	1–2	1–4	0–2	
Aromatic hydro-carbons§	Sy, S	1–2	1–3	0	Anesthetic
Halogenated hydro-carbons//	Sy	1–3	0	0	Anesthetic
Alcohols, ethers, others	Sy, E, S, URT	1–2	1–4	0–2	Anesthetic
Group IV					
Inorganic and organo-metallic gases	Lung parenchyma	1–2	0–3	0–2	

*Symbols used for corrosive and toxic effects
  Sy = systemic
  E   = eyes
  S   = skin
  URT = upper respiratory tract
†For explanation of the hazard rating system (0–4), see Hazard Identification System.
‡Methane, ethane, propane, butane, hexene, ethylene
§Toluene, xylene
//Chloroform, carbon tetrachloride, chlorobromomethane, Halon 1301, Halon 1211
  Sodeman TM: Clinical laboratory safety. Lab Med 11, No. 8:1980.

(Table 3-5; see Definitions of Flammables, and Classification of Flammable and Combustible Liquids). However, it is the *vapor* from the evaporation of a flammable (or combustible) liquid exposed to air or under the influence of heat, rather than the liquid itself, that burns (or explodes) in the presence of a source of ignition. This flammable vapor–air mixture spreads readily and the vapor trail can be ignited and will continue to burn or explode (see Table 3-6). The point at which a flammable or combustible liquid gives off enough vapor to form an

Table 3-5. Flammable Liquids Commonly Used in the Laboratory

FLAMMABLE LIQUID	FLASH POINT (°F)	IGNITION TEMPERATURE (°F)	TOXICITY*	HAZARD IDENTIFICATION†		
				HEALTH	FLAMMABILITY	REACTIVITY
Hydrocarbons						
Toluene	40	896	Sy	2	3	0
Isopentane (2-methylbutane)	<−60	788	Sy	1	4	0
Xylene	81	986	S, URT	2	3	0
Petroleum ether (benzene)	0	550	Sy, S, URT	1	4	0
Alcohols						
Methyl alcohol (methanol)	52	725	Sy, E, S, URT	1	3	0
Ethyl alcohol (ethanol)	55	689	Sy, E, URT	0	3	0
Isopropyl alcohol (2-propanol)	53	750	Sy, E	1	3	0
Tertiary butyl alcohol	52	896	S, URT	1	3	0
Glycerine (glycerol)	320	698		1	1	0
Ketones						
Acetone (2-propanone)	0	869	S	1	3	0
Methyl isobutyl ketone	73	860	Sy, E, URT	2	3	0
Esters						
Ethyl acetate	24	800	Sy, E, URT	1	3	0
Amyl acetate	77	680	URT	1	3	0
Isoamyl acetate	77	680	Sy	1	3	0

(continued)

Table 3-5. Flammable Liquids Commonly Used in the Laboratory (continued)

FLAMMABLE LIQUID	FLASH POINT (°F)	IGNITION TEMPERATURE (°F)	TOXICITY*	HAZARD IDENTIFICATION†		
				HEALTH	FLAMMABILITY	REACTIVITY
Glycols						
Ethylene glycol	232	752	Sy	1	1	0
Propylene glycol	210	700	S	0	1	0
Dioxane	54	356	Sy, E, URT	2	3	0
Chloro-compounds						
1,2-Dichloroethane	56	775	Sy, E, URT	2	3	0
Ether	−49	320	Sy	2	4	0
Amines						
Diethylamine	0	594	S	2	3	0
Cyclohexanes						
Cyclohexanol	154	572	Sy	1	2	0
Cyclohexanone	111	788	E, URT	1	2	0
Aldehydes						
Acetaldehyde	−36	347	Sy, S	2	4	2

*Symbols used for corrosive and toxic effects
Sy = systemic
E   = eyes
S   = skin
URT = upper respiratory tract
†For explanation of the hazard rating system (0–4), see Hazard Identification System.
Sodeman TM: Clinical laboratory safety. Lab Med 11, No. 8:1980.

ignitable mixture with air and produce a flame is called the *flash point* of the liquid. When a source of ignition is present, liquids having flash points *below* room temperature (*e.g.,* acetone) may be hazardous even at room temperature. As a general rule, whenever it can be avoided, do *not* use low–flash point liquids.

Liquids with flash points *higher* than room temperature become dangerous when heated. The rate of vaporization of a liquid depends on its vapor pressure and temperature; the vaporization rate increases with increased temperatures. Flammable liquids are thus a greater fire hazard at higher temperatures than are combustible liquids, which are not quite as dangerous.

(Text continues on p. 68)

Table 3-6. Flash Points of the Flammable and Combustible Solvents Used in the Laboratory

SOLVENT	FLASH POINT (°F)
Acetone	0
Acetic acid	109
Acetic anhydride	129
Amyl acetate	77
Amyl alcohol	91
Butyl alcohol	82
Butyl ether	40
Benzene	12
Carbon disulfide	−22
Cyclohexane	− 4
Diethylamine	−15
Dioxane	54
Ethanol	55
Ether (diethyl or ethyl)	−49
Ether alcohol	Depends on ratio
Ethyl acetate	24
Ethylene chloride (dichloride)	56
Heptane	25
Hexane	− 7
Isoamyl alcohol (isopentyl alcohol)	109
Isooctate	56
Isopropanol	53
Methyl alcohol	52
Methylal	0
Methylethyl ketone	20
2-octanol (capryl alcohol)	140
Pentane	−56
Pentyl acetate (amyl acetate)	77
Petroleum ether	−70
n-propyl alcohol	77
Pyridine	68
Tetrahydrofuran	6
Toluene	40
Xylene	81

(Adapted from Henry, RJ: Safety in the Clinical Laboratory. Van Nuys, CA, BioScience Enterprises, 1976)

DEFINITIONS—FLAMMABLES

Flash point of a liquid is the temperature at which it gives off vapors sufficient to form an ignitible mixture with the air near the surface of the liquid.

Flammable liquids are those having a flash point below 140°F.

Combustible liquids have a flash point at or above 140°F.

Liquefied compressed gases are flammable liquids with a vapor pressure above forty pounds per square inch absolute at 100°F.

Ignition temperature (autoignition temperature) of a substance is the minimum temperature required to initiate or cause self-sustained combustion without ignition from an external energy source.

The lower flammable limit (lower explosive limit) is the minimum concentration of vapor in air below which a flame is *not* propagated when an ignition source is present. Below this concentration, the mixture is too lean to burn.

The upper flammable limit (upper explosive limit) is the maximum concentration of vapor in air in which a flame can be propagated. Above this concentration, the mixture is too rich to burn.

Flammable range consists of all concentrations between the lower flammable limit and the upper flammable limit.

Specific gravity of a liquid is the ratio of its density to that of water under specified conditions. This term is important in that a material that does not mix with water will float if its specific gravity is less than 1 and will sink and be covered with water if its specific gravity is greater than 1.

Vapor density is expressed as the relative density of a vapor with respect to air at the same temperature. Thus, a vapor having a density less than 1 will tend to rise, and a vapor with a density greater than 1 will tend to sink.

Water solubility is sometimes important in determining whether water can be effectively used to flush away flammable liquids. Remember that a water solution of soluble solvents can give off sufficient vapors to burn. For example, a 5 percent solution of ethyl alcohol in water has a determinable flash point.

From *Guide for Safety in the Chemical Laboratory* by the Manufacturing Chemists Association Copyright © 1972 by Van Nostrand Reinhold Company. Reprinted by permission of the publisher.

CLASSIFICATION OF FLAMMABLE
AND COMBUSTIBLE LIQUIDS

The following classification system for flammable and combustible liquids (from NFPA 321) is based on the division of liquids that will burn into three categories. It is anticipated that in most areas the indoor temperature could reach 100°F at some time during the year. Therefore, all liquids with flash points below 100°F are called Class I liquids. In some areas the ambient temperature could exceed 100°F, or only a moderate degree of heating would be required to heat the liquid to its flash point. Based on this concept, an arbitrary division of 100°F to 140°F was established for liquids in this flash point range, to be known as Class II liquids. Since liquids with flash points higher than 140°F would require considerable heating from a source other than ambient temperatures, they have been identified as Class III liquids.

Flammable Liquids

Flammable liquids have flash points below 100°F and vapor pressures not exceeding 40 psia at 100°F.

Class I liquids include those with flash points below 100°F and may be subdivided as follows:

Class IA includes those with flash points below 73°F and with boiling points below 100°F.

Class IB includes those with flash points below 73°F and with boiling points at or above 100°F.

Class IC includes those flash points at or above 73°F and below 100°F.

Combustible Liquids

Liquids with flash points at or above 100°F are referred to as combustible liquids and may be subdivided as follows:

Class II liquids have flash points at or above 100°F and below 140°F.

Class IIIA liquids have flash points at or above 140°F and below 200°F.

Class IIIB liquids have flash points at or above 200°F.

Underwriters Laboratories Inc., Classification

Underwriters Laboratories Inc., has a classification system for grading the relative flammability hazards of various liquids, based on the following scale:

Ether class 100
Gasoline class 90–100
Alcohol (ethyl) class 60–70
Kerosene class* 30–40
Paraffin oil class 10–20

*A standard kerosene of 100°F closed cap flash point is rated 40.

The flash point, although the commonly accepted and most important criterion of the relative hazard of flammable and combustible liquids, is by no means the only factor in evaluating the hazard. The ignition temperature, flammable range, rate of evaporation, reactivity when contaminated or exposed to heat, density, and rate of diffusion of the vapor are also important factors. After the fire has burned for a short time, however, these other factors have comparatively little influence on its burning characteristics.

Flammables and Combustibles

Flammable and combustible liquids are ubiquitous in the laboratory. For this reason, medical technologists should be thoroughly familiar with the subject of flammables and the physical properties (flammability characteristics) of each solvent used in the laboratory. It should be noted that these same flammables may also be corrosive and toxic (see listing below) and handled accordingly.

TOXIC AND FLAMMABLE CHEMICALS*

TOXIC TO SKIN	TOXIC THROUGH INHALATION	FLAMMABLE OR EXPLOSIVE
Acetic acid		
Acetone	Acetone	Acetone
Acetyl chloride	Ammonia	Amyl alcohol
Alkali, caustic	Amyl alcohol	Benzene
Aniline	Aniline	Butyl acetate
Bromine	Benzene	Butyl alcohol
Carbon disulfide	Bromine	Carbon disulfide
Chromic acid	Butyl acetate	Cellosolve
Chloroform	Butyl alcohol	Cellosolve
Cresol	Carbon disulfide	acetate
Ethylene oxide	Carbon dioxide	Chloroform
Hydrochloric acid	(dry ice)	Dichlorethylene
Hydrofluoric acid	Carbon tetra-	Ethyl acetate
Hydrogen peroxide	chloride	Ethyl alcohol
(30%)	Chlorine	Ethyl chloride

*Adapted with permission from A Laboratory Safety Guide (Rev) 1980. California Association of Public Health Laboratory Directors, California State Department of Health Services, 1980.

TOXIC TO SKIN	TOXIC THROUGH INHALATION	FLAMMABLE OR EXPLOSIVE
Iodine		
Mercuric chloride	Chloroform	Ethyl ether
Nitrobenzene	Cresol	Ethylene dichloride
Nitric acid	Dichlorethylene	Ethylene oxide
Perchloric acid	Ethyl chloride	Formic acid
Phenol	Ethyl ether	Hexane
Silver nitrate	Ethylene dich-	Methyl alcohol
Sodium Hydroxide	loride	Perchloric acid
Sodium hypo-	Formaldehyde	Toluene (toluol)
chlorite (bleach)	Formic acid	Trichlorethylene
Sulfuric acid	Hydrochloric acid	Xylene (xylol)
Trichlorethylene	(fumes)	
Tricresol	Hydrogen sulfide	
Xylene (xylol)	Hydrofluoric acid	
	Mercury	
	Methyl alcohol	
	Methylene chloride	
	Nitrobenzene	
	Nitric acid	
	Tetrachlorethylene	
	Toluene (toluol)	
	Xylene (xylol)	

For working with flammables, protective clothing is recommended. Minimal amounts of the flammables are to be kept in the working area and these only in approved cans and cabinets (Table 3-7). No flames or ignition sources of any sort are allowed where flammables are in use or stored. Flammable liquids should be well labeled with both *FLAM-MABLE* and *DANGER* signs and also used and stored where ventilation is good. Refrigerated flammables may be stored only in explosion-proof refrigerators. Flammables should be heated only with hot water, steam, or an electric mantle. They should not be stored in glass containers on high shelves and must not be stored or transferred near an exit. Approved metal safety cans are best for transporting flammable solvents but, when glass is required for purity, cushioned safety carriers are necessary.

Accidents involving flammables necessitate prompt and appro-

Table 3-7. Maximum Allowable Size of Containers and Portable Tanks

CONTAINER TYPE	FLAMMABLE LIQUIDS			COMBUSTIBLE LIQUIDS	
	Class IA	Class IB	Class IC	Class II	Class III
Glass	1 pt	1 qt	1 gal	1 gal	5 gal
Metal (other than DOT drums) or approved plastic	1 gal	5 gal	5 gal	5 gal	5 gal
Safety cans	2 gal	5 gal	5 gal	5 gal	5 gal
Metal drum (DOT spec)	60 gal	60 gal	60 gal	60 gal	60 gal
Approved portable tanks	660 gal	660 gal	660 gal	660 gal	660 gal
Polyethylene DOT Spec 34, or as authorized by DOT exemption	1 gal	5 gal	5 gal	60 gal	60 gal

SI Units: 1 pt = 0.473 liters; 1 qt = 0.95 liters; 1 gal = 3.785 liters.
Reprinted with permission from NFPA 30-1981, Flammable and Combustible Liquids Code, Copyright © 1980, National Fire Protection Association, Quincy, MA 02269. This reprinted material is not the complete and official position of the NFPA on the referenced subject which is represented only by the standard in its entirety.

priate attention. When a spill occurs on the skin, rinse the area well. If a flammable is accidentally ingested, induce vomiting with syrup of ipecac. If a person's clothing should catch fire, smother the fire with a fire blanket and get medical help immediately. Do not clean the skin with solvents. Any spill rags used for cleanup should be immediately placed into safety cans.

In transferring one flammable (solvent) in a metal container to another metal container, a voltage potential is created and, under these conditions, a static spark can cause ignition. If two containers are metal, they must, therefore, be bonded before pouring. Metal-to-metal contact is essential and so dirt, paint, rust and so on must be removed from the contact points. Bonding is not necessary if one container is glass.

Plastic containers are sometimes used to avoid the breakage problems that occur with glass containers and the contamination problems that occur with metal containers. Plastic containers must be chosen with particular attention to their compatibility with the contained liquid. For example, polyethylene containers are generally unsuitable for aldehydes, ketones, esters, higher-molecular-weight alcohols, benzene, toluene, various oils, silicone fluids, and halogenated hydrocarbons. Thus, in order to avoid this incompatibility, labels on plastic containers should indicate the container's constituent materials as well as the chemicals contained.

Toxic Substances

Toxic substances (also called poisons) in relatively small quantities can cause illness or death when ingested (lead, mercury), inhaled (fumes, gases, vapors), or absorbed through the skin. The numerous toxic chemicals used in the laboratory are toxic only in their free or chemically available forms. Toxicity of these chemicals *in vivo* is dependent on their absorption and distribution (protein binding, transformation, storage, excretion) tolerance and rate of metabolism (Fig. 3-4). Toxic effects may be categorized as *local* or *systemic* or *acute* or *chronic*. Exposures are usually termed *acute* or *chronic*. Containers of toxics should be labeled with both a *DANGER* and a *TOXIC* label and toxic chemicals should always be handled under a hood. If the toxicity of a substance is not known, treat it as if it were toxic. Also remember that toxics may be flammable and may be explosion hazards as well.

Whenever possible, substitute less hazardous materials for toxic ones. As a preventive measure, use protective clothing and hoods when working with toxic substances. Get medical help or advice if prolonged or unexpected contact with a toxic substance occurs. Thorough washing after the use of toxic chemicals is mandatory, as is medical surveillance at regular intervals (Table 3-8).

Maximum allowable safe-exposure limits to toxic materials have been developed from the best available data reflecting the human health effects of these toxic materials. They are called *Threshold Limit Values* (TLVs). These values, being averages, however, do not reflect individual sensitivities. TLVs are used by the federal government to set a safe-exposure level for a majority of those who receive occupational exposure to toxic materials. Regular measurements and monitoring of

the contaminant level in the workplace reduces the likelihood that
employees will be exposed in excess of the TLV (Table 3-9).

Permissible Exposure Limit (PEL) is a term closely related to
TLV. It is used in the OSHA standards to describe the level and duration of allowable employee exposures to the OSHA-regulated toxic
chemicals.

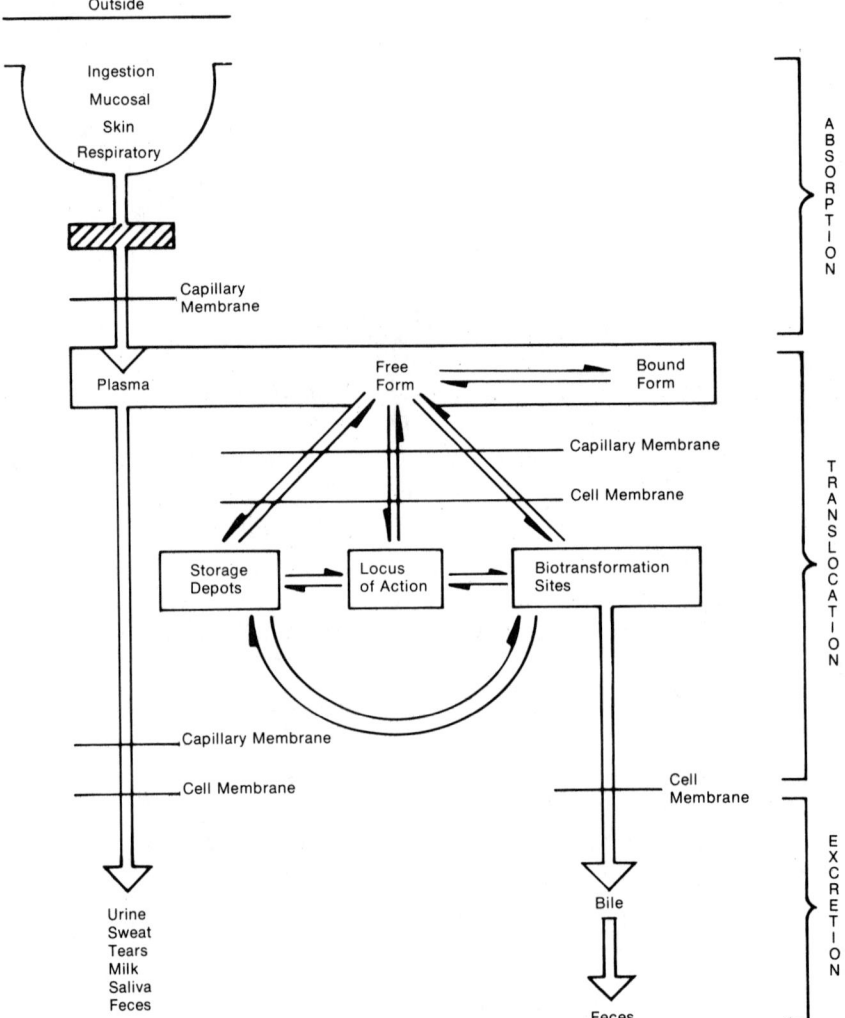

Fig. 3-4. Fate of chemicals in the body.

Table 3-8. Potential Effects of Some Laboratory Chemicals

AGENT	EFFECT
Sulfur dioxide	Extremely toxic; severe burns to lungs
Carbon disulfide	Irritates skin, eyes, nose, respiratory tract; high concentrations affect nervous system causing unconsciousness and even death
Nitrogen	Can asphyxiate because it reduces oxygen in air; termed "asphyxiating gas"
Carbon tetrachloride	Damaging to liver even at exposure level with no discernible odor
Hydrogen cyanide	Absorbed through skin easily; most rapidly acting of all known poisons
Hydrogen sulfide	Can desensitize sense of smell and irritate respiratory tract; concentrations above 700 ppm cause breathing to stop
Carbon monoxide	Prevents oxygenation of blood
Nitric acid	Can produce lung edema, eventually suffocating victim from fluid accumulation
Trichloroacetic acid	Very severe caustic; respiratory-tract irritant
Acetic acid	Severely caustic; chronic exposure to vapor can lead to chronic bronchitis
Benzidine	Absorbed rapidly through skin; salts can cause cancer
Phenol	Corrosive to skin; contact dermatitis even from dilute solutions
Ethers	Depression of central nervous system
Benzene	Acts on bone marrow to destroy production of blood cells associated with some leukemias

Roach GC: Laboratory Safety: Principles for Personal Practice. Houston, American Society for Medical Technology, 1978. Reprinted with permission.

Table 3-9. Threshold Limit Values for Some Common Laboratory Chemicals

SUBSTANCE	PARTS PER MILLION	mg/m^3
Acetic acid	10	25
Acetone	1000	3400
Butyl acetate (*n*-butyl acetate)	150	710
Butyl alcohol	100	300
Chloroform (trichlormethane)	50	240
Cyclohexane	300	1050
Diethylamine	25	75
Diozane (diethylemedioxide) skin	100	360
Ethyl acetate	400	1400
Ethyl alcohol (ethanol)	1000	1900
Ethyl ether	400	1200
Heptane (*n*-heptane)	500	2000
Isoamyl alcohol	100	360
Isobutyl alcohol	100	300
Isopropyl alcohol	400	980
Methyl alcohol (methanol)	200	260
Nitric acid	2	5
Nitrobenzene (skin)	1	5
Nitrogen, dioxide	5	9
Oxalic acid		1
Phenol (skin)	5	19
Phosphoric acid		1
Picric acid (skin)		.1
Selenium compounds (as Se)		.2
Sodium hydroxide		2
Sulfuric acid		1
O-Toluidize (skin)	5	22
Xylene (xylol)	100	435

Roach GC: Laboratory Safety: Principles for Personal Practice. Houston, American Society for Medical Technology, 1978. Reprinted with permission.

Mercury

Metallic mercury and its compounds can be absorbed into the body by inhalation, by ingestion, or through the skin. Poisonous effects develop very slowly unless large doses in compound or vapor form are absorbed over a short time. A major concern with metallic mercury is its high volatility, and this increases greatly after spills because of the vast increase in surface area. Spilled mercury, with insidious poisonous vapors, presents an extremely difficult cleanup problem and should be removed only with special aspirators or mercury vacuums. Powdered sulfur can be used on spilled mercury and swept up 24 hours later as mercury sulfide. Elemental mercury should be kept in tightly closed containers or stored under water. From a breakage aspect, polyethylene storage containers are safer than glass containers. In any case, mercury should not come into direct contact with the skin.

Mercury (elemental or compounds) should not be flushed down drains but instead can be precipitated with sodium chloride and discarded with solid wastes. Mercury should be used only in well-ventilated areas. OSHA has defined a ceiling concentration for mercury of 0.1 mg/m^3 of air. Some mercury compounds may also pose serious reactivity problems. Nitric acid and ethyl alcohol react with mercury to form a highly explosive mercury fulminate.

Benzene

Benzene, a particularly dangerous solvent, exerts its toxic actions primarily on the blood-forming organs, especially the liver and kidneys. It is now considered a carcinogen by OSHA (see Appendix A). Inhalation of relatively small amounts of benzene over long periods of time may result in chronic poisoning; contact of benzene with the skin may result in skin absorption. Benzene is also a very flammable solvent and requires special handling and disposal. Substitute other products for benzene whenever possible, although these may also pose their own hazards (*e.g.,* 1, 1, 1 trichlorethane, acetone, toluene).

Explosives

Explosives include materials that, under certain conditions of temperature, shock, or chemical reaction, can decompose rapidly to evolve either large volumes of gas or so much heat that the surrounding air is forced to expand very rapidly, resulting in an explosion. As a general rule, all flammable chemicals such as organic compounds must be kept away from oxidizing agents (*e.g.,* acids). Those materials with flash points at or below room temperature should be considered extremely dangerous. Those chemicals that can accumulate in dust form represent a relatively high to medium explosion hazard and those that, by chemical reaction, can support or initiate an explosion are classified as medium to low explosion hazards. However, these are only general designations. *Explosive* primarily defines a set of conditions, not a chemical type. Most explosives will also be found under other hazards categories as well. Take special care with the following chemicals, which have explosive potential:

Acetone
Benzene
Butyl acetate
Butyl alcohol
Carbon disulfide
Ethyl acetate
Ethyl alcohol
Ethyl ether
Gasoline
Methanol
N-Amyl acetate
Amyl alcohol
Toluene
Xylene
Picric acid

Picric Acid

For safety in transport, picric acid is often provided with 10% to 20% water added. In the dry state, picric acid poses an extreme explosion hazard if not stored properly because it is highly sensitive to shock. Over time, it will change from a solution to a crystalline state. It should be stored in an inverted position to prevent drying in the area of the bottle cap or it may detonate when the cap is unscrewed. Old picric acid on a storage-room shelf should not go unnoticed or it may require a bomb squad for safe removal.

Perchloric Acids

Perchloric acid, although it can be a respiratory irritant, is primarily an explosion hazard. It explodes on contact with reducing agents and organic materials and must not be used on wooden workbenches. Dry perchloric acid becomes extremely explosive. As a result of the use of improper hoods for perchloric-acid work (*e.g.,* protein-bound iodine test [PBI]), several explosions have resulted during cleaning of the hood blowers, drains, and so on. A hazard persists in all these former-PBI laboratories if the ductwork has not been properly washed. Specially designed hoods with water washdown and noncombustible construction are mandatory for perchloric-acid procedures. Perchloric-acid distillations should be avoided if possible; if this is not possible, suitable hoods with safety shields are the only acceptable workspace.

Perchloric acid should be kept on glass trays with enough volume to contain the acid in case of a spill. Discolored acid must be disposed of immediately after gentle dilution in a beaker with several volumes of cold water. Organic matter must be digested with nitric acid *before* the addition of perchloric acid.

Oxidizers

Oxidizers are materials that contain oxygen available to react with reducing materials to yield an overall net energy release. (A few materials containing *no* oxygen are also classed as oxidizers.) Generally, the following chemical types are oxidizers: compounds ending in -*ite* or -*ate* or with the prefix *per-*, *oxoacids*, peroxides, halogens, halogen-nitrogen reacted compounds, and reacted mixed halogens.

It is the unplanned or greater than expected, often explosive, energy release of some oxidizers that poses so very serious a hazard. Containers of oxidizers should be labeled both *DANGER* and *OXIDIZER*. If possible, work with oxidizers should be performed in a hood with the sash lowered. The technician should wear protective clothing when working with oxidizers. Hydrocarbon greases or oils must *never* be used with oxygen or halogens.

Peroxide-Forming Compounds

The class of oxidizers that is of most concern in the laboratory, because of its extreme instability, is that of the organic peroxides. Organic peroxides have extreme sensitivity to shock, sparks, heat, friction, impact, light, strong oxidizers, reducers, and other forms of accidental ignition. Peroxides have a specific rate of decomposition under any given set of conditions. All peroxides are extremely flammable.

Common peroxide-forming solvents are ethers, acetals, ureas, amides, lactams, aldehydes, and vinyl monomers that polymerize. Generally, pure compounds are *more* subject to peroxide buildup. The more volatile compounds are greater hazards because the peroxide becomes concentrated as evaporation occurs.

Package sizes of peroxide formers must be limited. Storage time should be limited to 3 months after opening unless the contents are tested and shown to be free of peroxides. All peroxide formers must be sealed to prevent contact with air and must be stored away from heat and light. Flashproof refrigerated space maintained solely for peroxides is the preferred method of storage.

The following general precautions should be read and followed for all peroxide-forming compounds. In addition, laboratories may have their own specific techniques and regulations about handling of these chemicals, which may add to or modify the general precautions presented here.

General Instructions and Precautions for Handling Peroxides

Limit the quantity of peroxide to the minimum amount required. Do not return the unused peroxide to the original container. Clean up all peroxide spills immediately. Solutions of peroxides can be absorbed with vermiculite. The sensitivity of most peroxides to shock and heat can be reduced by diluting with an inert solvent such as benzene and aliphatic hydrocarbons. Toluene is known to decompose diacyl peroxides. (Addition of inhibitors must not *ever* be initiated by an uninstructed medical technologist.) Do not use solutions of peroxides in volatile solvents under conditions in which the solvent will be vaporized, thereby increasing the peroxide concentration in the solution. Never use a metal spatula with peroxides, because contamination by metals can lead to explosive combinations; instead use ceramic or wooden spatulas.

Smoking, open flames, and other sources of heat are not permitted near peroxides. Friction, grinding, and all forms of impact must be avoided, especially with solid peroxides. Use polyethylene bottles with screw-cap lids, not glass containers with screw-cap lids or glass stoppers. To minimize the rate of decomposition, peroxides should be stored at the lowest possible temperatures consistent with solubility or freezing point. *Caution*—Do not refrigerate liquid or solutions of peroxides at or below the temperature at which the peroxide freezes or precipitates because peroxides in these forms are extremely shock and heat sensitive.

Disposal of peroxides. Caution—Never dispose of pure peroxides. Peroxides must be diluted.

- *Small quantities* (25 g or less) of peroxides can be disposed of by being first diluted with water to a concentration of 2% or less and then transferred to a polyethylene disposal bottle containing an aqueous solution of a reducing agent (*e.g.,* ferrous sulfate or sodium bisulfite). The material is then handled as is any other waste chemical for disposal but must *not* be mixed with other chemicals. Spilled peroxides should be absorbed on vermiculite as quickly as possible. The vermiculite–peroxide mixture may then be burned directly or stirred with a suitable solvent to form a slurry, which can then be treated as just described. *Caution*— Never flush organic peroxides down the drain.
- *Large quantities* (25 g or more) of peroxide require special planning before the material is prepared or purchased. Planning must include intended handling, storage, and disposal procedures, which are determined by the physical and chemical properties of the particular peroxide.

Ethers

Ethers are a class of chemicals that presents several types of hazard in the laboratory—they are highly flammable, may cause physical disorders, and easily form explosive peroxides. The ether of most concern in the clinical laboratory is ethyl ether. Ethyl ether has a flash point of $-45°C$ and at room temperature gives off vapors that can be ignited by an open flame, a spark, or static electricity. All ether work should be conducted in a fume hood. Ether should always be stored in safety containers.

Ethers are included in this section because of their ability to form extremely explosive peroxides. Ethers, especially cyclic ethers and ethers containing primary and secondary alcohol groups, are peroxide formers. It is the chemical reaction of ether and oxygen that causes the explosive peroxide formation. The rate of peroxide formation depends on the particular ether and the storage conditions (*e.g.,* exposure to air or sunlight). Storing ether in refrigerators, especially the nonexplosion-proof type, creates a further danger. Refrigeration does not prevent peroxide formation, nor does it prevent vaporization. As a result, dangerous quantities of vapor may collect inside the refrigerator and be ignited by any spark. Ether is best stored in a sparkfree, continuously vented fume hood or well-ventilated shelf. The amount of ether stored should be as small as possible. The length of storage time should be short, depending on the type of ether (1 month to 6 months for an opened can and no more than 1 year for an unopened can). Containers of ethyl or isopropyl ether should be labeled with the date when they are opened. Ethers are packaged in an air atmosphere and will form peroxides whether the container has been opened or not. Peroxide inhibitors may be added to some ethers, but this may be done only by the manufacturer, not by the medical technologist. Ether should not be stored in glass containers.

EQUIPMENT—AN APPROACH TO SAFE USE

An extensive array of instruments is available for use in the clinical laboratory, and the sophistication and choices continue to grow. Along with this growth come additional safety codes and regulations for the manufacture and use of these products. The net effect is to make the laboratory a safer place to work and to provide the patient with an increasing number of highly accurate test results. Regular inspection and maintenance and mandatory adherence to standard operating procedures are required in the care and use of *all* laboratory equipment. Unmodified homemade equipment, improper maintenance, improvised procedures, and poor housekeeping present unacceptable risks to machines, technicians, and patients. Although pertinent reminders are presented here on the safe use of some major pieces of clinical-chemistry equipment, this is not intended as a substitute for thorough instruction on each instrument when it is first used. Computers and automated chemistry analysis instruments are beyond the scope and intent of this volume.

Autoclaves

Because autoclaves present a significant safety hazard, owing to both high heat and high pressure, the medical technologist should be thoroughly trained in their operation. Although reminders are included here for safe operating techniques, thorough hands-on training is the only satisfactory learning device for autoclave operation.

Autoclave Safety Reminders

- Make sure the temperature and pressure are back to normal before opening an autoclave.
- Use heat-resistant gloves when putting items into or removing items from an autoclave. (Be careful—steam *can* penetrate heat-resistant gloves.)
- Loosen caps of any containers to prevent explosions, boil-overs, and implosions in the autoclave.
- Be cautious in autoclaving plastic materials.
- *Never* autoclave solvents.
- Keep your face well away from the door when opening a hot autoclave.
- Follow the *specific* manufacturer's directions for each type of autoclave.
- See the section on autoclaves in Chapter 6.

Stirrers, Shakers, and Evaporators

Stirring and mixing devices are often used in procedures performed under the laboratory hood. They must not produce sparks in the hood and should have off/on controls located outside the hood in case conditions require shutdown with the hood sash closed. The devices must be used only in the manner prescribed by the manufacturer.

Centrifuges

Accidents in and with centrifuges can be expected in the laboratory because the centrifuge is such an integral part of so many laboratory procedures. Proper precautions and knowledge can help to limit centrifuge accidents to those caused by mechanical faults rather than human error.

Centrifuges must never be operated with the cover open. Most centrifuges are now built with this safety feature included and will not function when open. Centrifuge operators should be extra cautious with long hair, beards, ribbons, jewelry, and loose clothing because of the serious consequences of becoming entangled.

Uncapped tubes can create a large volume of aerosols and, therefore, all tubes of specimens and flammables should be covered with caps or parafilm. Carrier cups must be kept clean and smooth. Regular professional maintenance of the centrifuge is important. If an unusual noise is heard during centrifugation, the centrifuge should be stopped and the load checked for balance and breakage. Depending on the contents, it may be preferable to let any aerosol settle before opening the centrifuge after stopping it if the sound of breaking glass is heard. All centrifuge tubes should be checked for stress lines before they are used. Tubes used in angle-head centrifuges should never be filled so that the liquid may be in contact with the lip of the tube. This is true of centrifuging of all hazardous substances.

Safety Cabinets

Safety cabinets designed to hold flammables should be marked *FLAMMABLES STORAGE* and include a *KEEP FIRE AWAY* warning in large letters on the front of the cabinet. They are made with removable plugs designed for venting to prevent vapor accumulation. These plugs must be left in place unless the cabinet is hooked up to a ventilation system. Safety cabinets are constructed of fire-resistant materials. All of the stored contents must be well labeled and dated and should be inventoried at least every 6 months. A list of contents should be available on or near the safety cabinet. The size of containers storing flammables must comply with fire safety codes (see Classification of Flammable and Combustible Liquids, earlier in this chapter). All containers must be kept tightly closed and incompatible chemicals must not be stored together (Tables 3-7, 3-10).

Safety cabinets are not for bulk storage. They are best used for storing the amount of flammables to be used weekly or daily. No more than three safety cabinets are allowed per laboratory module. A positive locking device is necessary for the door of the safety cabinet. Electrical grounding is not necessary. These cabinets should not be placed near tissue-processing equipment or other automated instruments using flammables.

Refrigerators

Laboratory refrigerators in routine operation do not present a hazard unless they are used improperly. The most dangerous type of improper use involves storing the wrong thing in the refrigerator. The best example of improper use is the storage of solvents in a regular refrigerator where vapors can accumulate and ignite. These materials can be stored safely only in an explosion-proof refrigerator that has *all* electrical contacts on the outside. Modifying a domestic refrigerator for safe chemical storage requires eliminating all lights, blowers, and electrical contacts from inside the box and having the door closure replaced with magnets. Drains in the bottom must be plugged as well to prevent spills and vapors from accidental contact with the motor.

All refrigerators must be properly labeled (Fig. 3-5). No food may be stored in chemical refrigerators. Material stored in refrigerators should be capped to be vaportight and spillproof. Uncapped or unlabeled containers are not allowed. Toxic or explosive material should not be placed in a laboratory refrigerator if this can be avoided. Dry ice should not be stored in walk-in refrigerators because it may become an asphyxiant if the carbon-dioxide level gets too high.

Heating Devices

Heating devices are used throughout the laboratory to sterilize, speed up reactions, produce separations, and perform other functions. It is obvious that proper maintenance and proper operation for all heating devices are mandatory (as they are for *all* laboratory equipment), but some specific additional precautions are included here.

In the laboratory, whenever possible, steam-heated devices rather than electrically heated devices should be used because their temperature never exceeds 100° C and there is no spark or shock hazard. All heating elements in any heating device must be enclosed by a nonconducting case that keeps "hot" wires separated from chemicals and technicians.

(Text continues on p. 86)

Table 3-10. List of Some Incompatible Chemicals

SUBSTANCES IN THE LEFT HAND COLUMN SHOULD BE STORED AND HANDLED SO THEY CANNOT POSSIBLY ACCIDENTALLY CONTACT CORRESPONDING SUBSTANCES IN THE RIGHT HAND COLUMN.

Alkaline and alkaline earth metals, such as sodium, potassium, cesium, lithium, magnesium, calcium, aluminum	Carbon dioxide, carbon tetrachloride, and other chlorinated hydrocarbons, any free acid or halogen. Do not use water, foam, or dry chemical on fires involving these metals.
Acetic acid	Chromic acid, nitric acid, hydroxyl-containing compounds, ethylene glycol, perchloric acid, peroxide, and permanganates
Acetone	Concentrated nitric and sulfuric acid mixtures
Acetylene	Chlorine, bromine, copper, silver, fluorine, and mercury
Ammonia (anhydrous)	Mercury, chlorine, calcium hypochlorite, iodine, bromine, and hydrogen fluoride
Ammonium nitrate	Acids, metal powders, flammable liquids, chlorates, nitrites, sulfur, finely divided organics or combustibles
Aniline	Nitric acid, hydrogen peroxide
Bromine	Ammonia, acetylene, butadiene, butane and other petroleum gases, sodium carbide, turpentine, benzene, and finely divided metals
Hydrofluoric acid, anhydrous (hydrogen fluoride)	Ammonia, aqueous or anhydrous
Hydrogen sulfide	Fuming nitric acid, oxidizing gases
Hydrocarbons (benzene, butane, propane, gasoline, turpentine)	Fluorine, chlorine, bromine, chromic acid, sodium peroxide
Iodine	Acetylene, ammonia (anhydrous or aqueous)
Mercury	Acetylene, fluminic acid ammonia
Nitric acid (concentrated)	Acetic acid, aniline, chromic acid, hydrocyanic acid, hydrogen sulfide, flammable liquids, flammable gases, and nitritable substances
Nitroparaffins	Inorganic bases
Oxygen	Oils, grease, hydrogen, flammable liquids, solids, or gases
Oxalic acid	Silver, mercury
Perchloric acid	Acetic anhydride, bismuth and its alloys, alcohol, paper, wood, grease, oils, organic amines or antioxidants.
Peroxides, organic	Acids (organic or mineral); avoid friction
Phosphorus (white)	Air, oxygen

Chemical	Keep out of contact with
Calcium carbide	Water (see also acetylene)
Calcium oxide	Water
Carbon, activated	Calcium hypochlorite
Copper	Acetylene, hydrogen peroxide
Chlorates	Ammonium salts, acids, metal powders, sulfur, finely divided organics or combustibles
Chromic acid	Acetic acid, naphthalene, camphor, glycerine, turpentine, alcohol, and other flammable liquids, paper, or cellulose
Chlorine	Ammonia, acetylene, butadiene, butane and other petroleum gases, hydrogen, sodium carbide, turpentine, benzene, and finely divided metals
Chlorine dioxide	Ammonia, methane, phosphine, and hydrogen sulfide
Fluorine	Isolate from everything
Hydrocyanic acid	Nitric acid, alkalis
Hydrogen peroxide	Copper, chromium, iron, most metals or their salts, any flammable liquid, combustible materials, aniline, nitromethane
Potassium chlorate	Acids (see also chlorate)
Potassium perchlorates	Acids (see also perchloric acid)
Potassium permanganate	Glycerine, ethylene glycol, benzaldehyde, any free acid
Silver	Acetylene, oxalic acid, tartaric acid, fulminic acid, ammonium compounds
Sodium	See alkaline metals (above)
Sodium nitrate	Ammonium nitrate and other ammonium salts
Sodium oxide	Water, any free acid
Sodium peroxide	Any oxidizable substance, such as ethanol, methanol, glacial acetic acid, acetic anhydride, benzaldehyde, carbon disulfide, glycerine, ethylene glycol, ethyl acetate, methyl acetate, and furfurol
Sulfuric acid	Chlorates, perchlorates, permanganates
Zirconium	Prohibit water, carbon tetrachloride, foam, and dry chemical on zirconium fires

Reprinted with permission from Safety Committee: Safety Handbook. Fairbanks, University of Alaska, 1977.

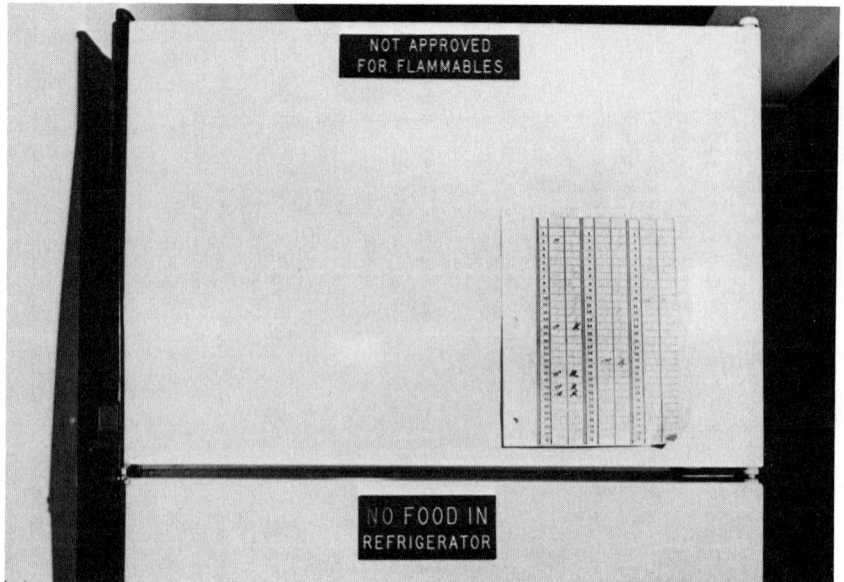

Fig. 3-5. All refrigerators must state plainly on the outside whether or not they are to be used for flammables.

Heating devices that may need to be left unattended for some time should be equipped with temperature sensing "fail-safe" devices, which switch off the equipment should a cooling-water or overheating accident occur.

Hot Plates

Only hot plates with enclosed heating elements should be used in laboratories. A hot plate that is cooling down should always bear a flag or marker to indicate that it may still be hot and should be avoided by other workers.

Bunsen Burners

If it is at all possible, open-flame Bunsen burners should *not* be used in the laboratory. If they must be used, they are *never* to be left burning unattended.

Oil Baths

Oil baths may be used when a small, oddly shaped vessel is being heated or when a constant temperature is needed. These should always have thermal sensing shutoff devices and thermometers. Care must be taken to avoid heating to the flash point of the oil being used.

Laboratory Ovens

Laboratory ovens may be used to remove solvents from other chemicals and to dry laboratory glassware. These ovens are usually not vented and, potentially, the volatized contents do escape into the laboratory air. Care, therefore, must be taken not to use a laboratory oven for drying volatile or toxic chemicals unless the oven is continuously vented. Only glassware rinsed with distilled water should be dried in a laboratory oven. Blowout vents are recommended for the back panels of laboratory ovens. Domestic ovens, unless modified electrically, should *not* be used in the laboratory.

Ventilation

Proper ventilation is a major concern for the laboratory from the aspects of both safety and comfort. Besides reducing the odors of chemicals and the heat generated by electronic equipment, ventilation also reduces the hazards of flammable and toxic substances in the air. Because the contents of laboratory air contain such a diversity of potential hazards, the air pressure in the laboratory should always be negative with respect to the adjoining corridors and the rest of the hospital building. This serves to draw the laboratory air out through the laboratory exhaust vents rather than into the hospital. Good laboratory ventilation, although essential, is not sufficient protection from toxic and flammable vapors that may be encountered by the laboratory worker. Procedures involving hazardous or volatile chemical manipulations, therefore, require the use of a hood. The chemicals themselves, when not in use, must be stored in vented safety cabinets. The hood exhaust should be chemically scrubbed or incinerated to avoid the release of high-level hazards to the outside environment.

Laboratory Hoods

Laboratory hoods are safety devices that are enclosed, except for necessary openings for exhaust purposes, on three sides and designed to draw air inward by means of mechanical ventilation. Laboratory hoods prevent toxic, flammable, or noxious vapors from entering the laboratory atmosphere, present a physical barrier from untoward chemical reactions, and serve to contain accidental spills. Because of their significant contribution to worker safety, hoods require certain essential maintenance and operating procedures. Hoods are only a secondary safety device, and cannot substitute for safe working procedures or chemical disposal. Hoods must always be evaluated before use to assure adequate face velocity, measured in linear feet per minute (fpm). Adequate face velocity is 60 fpm to 100 fpm, with 100 fpm preferred. The sash should be marked to show the maximum opening at which the hood face velocity meets the required air flow. Permanent stops should restrict closure so that, during work with flammables, enough air flow to prevent explosions is maintained. A continuous monitoring device for hood performance is recommended. The hood ports should be kept closed. Apparatus should be kept as far back in the hood as possible. Material should *not* be stored in the hood—the hood is often turned off and vapors can built up to dangerous or toxic levels (Fig. 3-6).

Mechanical ventilation must remain in operation at all times when hoods are in use, and for a sufficient time afterward, to clear the hood of airborne hazardous substances.

It is safer and less expensive to store chemicals in a vented safety cabinet than in a hood. The utility controls (gas, air, water, electricity) should be located outside of the hood (Fig. 3-7). The ventilation rates of all hoods should be measured, the data recorded, and the measurements kept for reference. The entire laboratory ventilation system should be routinely monitored to assure its efficiency for the safety of both the laboratory specifically and hospital generally.

Labeling

All containers of chemicals, whether in working use or storage, must be labeled to show the chemical identity, concentration, hazardous properties (if appropriate), and the dates of receipt and use. Safety cans

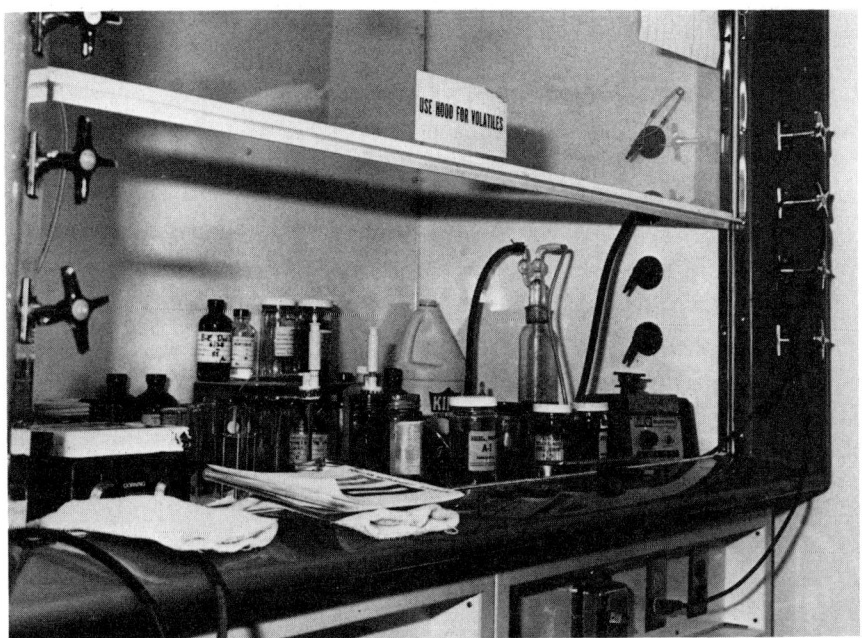

Fig. 3-6. The hood must not become a repository for abandoned hazardous chemicals.

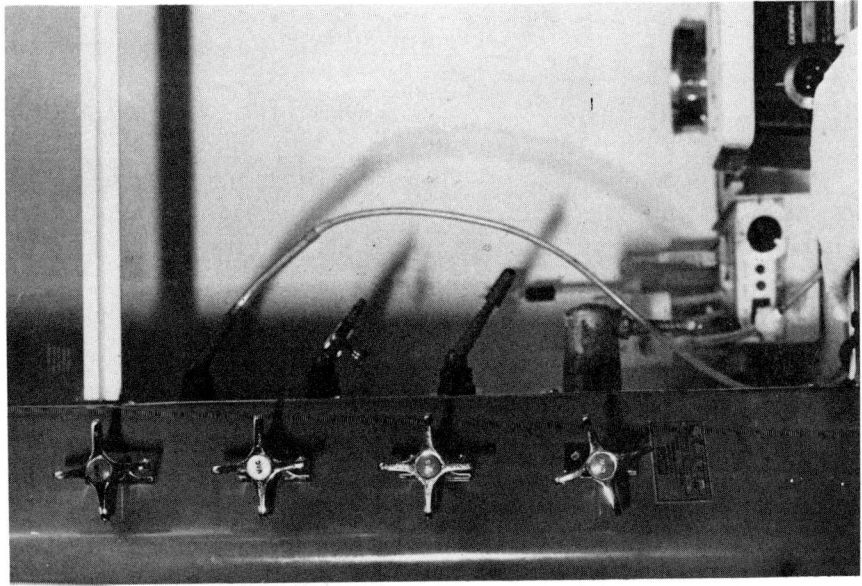

Fig. 3-7. Safety controls for air, gas, water, and so on should be available outside the hood, although outlets are inside the hood.

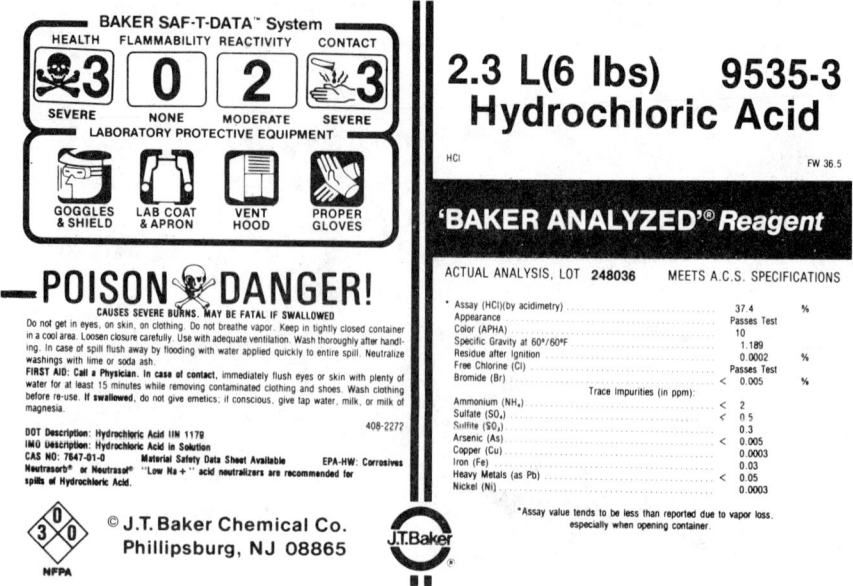

Fig. 3-8. Sample safety label. (Used with permission. Courtesy of J. T. Baker Chemical Co., Phillipsburg, NJ)

of stock chemicals may be labeled by name only. Materials having special hazards should always be so labeled (*e.g.,* poison, carcinogen).

Kits of chemical supplies are not exempt from these rules and the date the kit is put into service should be noted. All old labels must be removed before a container is relabeled. All labels must be read before a chemical is used and all those out of date should be discarded immediately through proper and appropriate disposal methods (Fig. 3-8).

Storage Areas

Although safety is a concern and a legal requirement throughout the clinical laboratory, an often forgotten source of danger is the storage area, especially one that is poorly planned and ill kept. This area, in a moderately sized laboratory, often contains large quantities of diverse liquid and solid chemicals of varying hazard, spare equipment, extra parts, assorted glassware, and a variety of poorly labeled and unclaimed bottles and cans. The sheer magnitude of its contents and the need to service so many laboratories and test procedures require strict order in the storeroom. This requirement addresses both functional and safety considerations. Luckily, laboratory inspections by fire marshals, accrediting bodies, and insurance examiners require certain basic standards in storage areas that otherwise might tend to become ignored.

The basic storeroom requirements—cool temperature, adequate ventilation, fire-resistant walls, sprinklers (or fire extinguishers), spark-proof lighting, and personnel-protective equipment—are mandated by laws and standards. Housekeeping, labeling, sizes of containers, and organization of stored contents are left to the laboratory staff (Fig. 3-9).

In determining where to store which chemicals in a storeroom, the particular hazards, reactivities, and incompatibilities of each chemical must be considered (Table 3-10 and list of Some Hazardous Substances). Alphabetical order is *not* a proper method of arrangement. The length of time chemicals are to be stored is also an important consideration because of decomposition, peroxide formation, and so on. A first-in, first-out system of reagent use is mandatory. In ordering chemicals, knowledge of the total amount of laboratory usage in a prescribed amount of time is essential because large quantities of little- or never-used chemicals present an unnecessary hazard. Most chemicals should be used or discarded within a limited period of time. Water-sensitive chemicals must be stored to prevent their accidental contact with water, which could then release hot and flammable or explosive gases. Obviously, water-reactive chemicals must not be stored under automatic sprinklers! Stock or often-used reagents should be stored within easy reach. Large containers should be stored near the floor, and corrosives should be placed in lead or plastic trays to hold the contents in case of leakage. Flammable liquids in quantities over 1 liter should be stored in metal safety cans or glass containers stored in trays. Depending on the quality and quantity of chemicals, fire safety cabinets should be used for flammable and dangerous chemicals. Special attention must be paid to heat sources in the storeroom—electrical sources, radiators, sunlight, and so on. Shelves should be equipped with a lip or restraints to prevent bottles from toppling or vibrating off. Apparatus and glass tubes should not project out from the shelves. No waste-paper accumulation or untidy housekeeping is allowed in the storeroom and, of course, the laboratorywide no-smoking restriction applies here as well. Chemicals must all be well and legibly labeled and inventoried

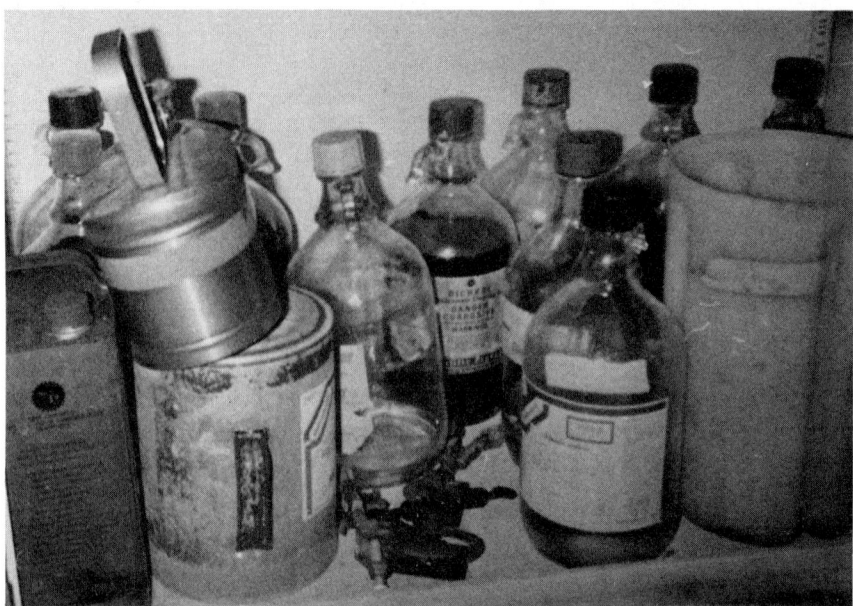

Fig. 3-9. Using an empty cabinet to store unwanted odds and ends represents a potential hazard and a safety violation.

regularly. Out-of-date chemicals must be discarded and dangerous chemicals (*e.g.,* peroxide formers) should be accessible for daily inspection. Chemicals may not be mixed or transferred to smaller containers in the storage area. It is essential that storeroom aisles to kept clear at all times to facilitate the use of the storeroom and to allow passage for personnel and equipment in an emergency.

Safety Labeling and the Right to Know

There is a growing awareness in the United States of the hazardous-substance exposure in many occupational categories. This awareness is due in large measure to the news media, government intervention, union demands, and progressive and concerned employers. At present, 23 states have enacted so called *right-to-know* laws, asserting that information on exposures, dangers, and suggested special handling be communicated to the affected worker. The clinical laboratory is one of these categories of employment. For many years, hospital-laboratory chemicals have carried such simple warning messages as *Flammable, Danger—Poison,* and *Warning—Corrosive Liquid* (Fig. 3-10). Although this does attract attention, it does not provide information about the level of danger or required special handling of the chemical contents. A literature search or consultation with a trained chemist would be necessary in most cases to uncover this vital safety information. Fortunately for the clinical-laboratory staff, a large commercial laboratory supplier, J. T. Baker Chemical Company, has introduced a novel labeling system called the BAKER SAF-T-DATA SYSTEM, incor-

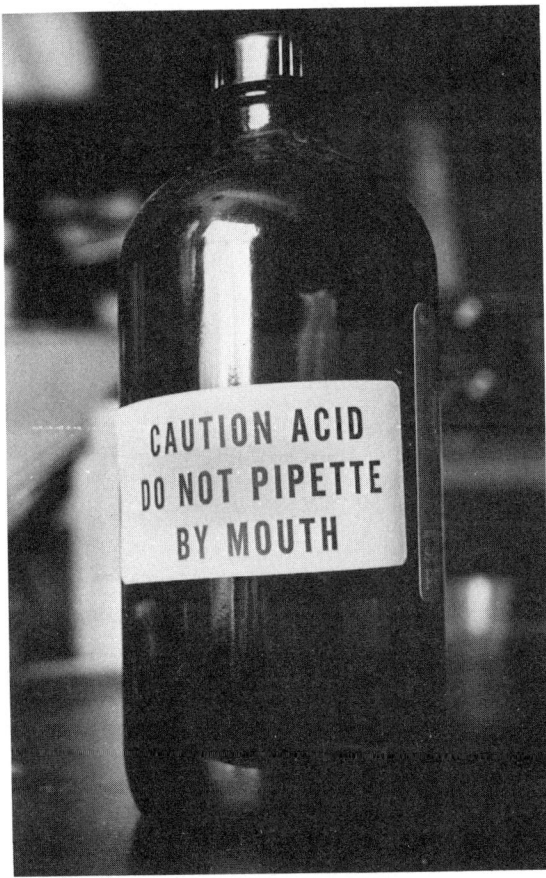

Fig. 3-10. With increased knowledge of laboratory hazards, a nondescriptive label such as this is no longer adequate to protect the worker.

porating hazard-classification criteria acceptable to the National Fire Protection Association (NFPA) and the National Institute for Occupational Safety and Health (NIOSH). This system is easy to understand, current with regulations, and communicated through the international language of colors, pictures, and numbers. It illustrates a complete and successful approach to providing the safety information required for clinical-laboratory exposure to hazardous chemicals.

Eventually, all 3000 J. T. Baker laboratory reagents will carry this SAF-T-DATA label (Fig. 3-8). The Baker system includes the following:

> A *numerical hazard code* (0–4) for each of four hazard categories: flammability, health, reactivity, and tissue contact
> A *hazard symbol code* to emphasize the dangers of substances rated 3 or 4
> A *storage color-coding system* to provide proper safe storage information; like colors can be stored together, and incompatible colors must be separated
> A *laboratory protective-equipment code* indicating the recommended basic personnel-protective clothing and equipment for using each chemical in a laboratory
> *The NFPA diamond*—a safety symbol, discussed previously, required by many municipal ordinances and intended to safeguard firefighters

Other information provided on the label includes the Department of Transportation (DOT) classification, the Environmental Protection Agency (EPA) hazardous-waste code, recommended spill-cleanup materials, the chemical abstract service (CAS) number, the availability of material safety data sheets, and the International Maritime Organization hazardous-waste data. It is likely that a labeling system such as this will eventually be used by all chemical companies in their further endeavors to protect occupational health and in addressing the right-to-know laws. The American Chemical Society considers the Baker system to be the most complete and informative one available and suggests it be a model for other suppliers to use.* Fisher Scientific has also introduced a new system called Fisher ChemAlert, which provides a similar, effective reagent label on Fisher chemicals.

(Text continues on p. 98)

*O'Neill GJ: Comment: A novel idea for communicating health and safety data. C&E News 27:1982

SOME HAZARDOUS SUBSTANCES

HAZARDOUS

Highly dangerous—will explode owing to heat, flame, shock

Acetylides
Acetyl peroxide
Aluminum alkyls
Ammonium chlorate
Diazoethane
Diazomethane
Dichloroacetylene
N,N′-diethyl carbanilide
Ethylene oxide
Formyl peroxide
Fulminates
Glycerol trinitrate
Hexane hexanitrate
Hydrogen (high pressure)
Hydrogen peroxide
  (<35% water)
Iodine azide
Lead azide
Manganese heptoxide
Mannitol hexanitrate
Mercury acetylide
Mercury azide
Methyl isocyanide
Nitrocellulose (dry)
Ozonides (dry)
Parathion
Perchloric acid
  (<10% water)
Phenyl diazosulfide
Picric acid and Cu, Pb, and
  Zn salts (dry)
Radioisotopes, gamma
  emitters
Silver azide
Tetracene
Tetracetylene dicarbonic acid
Tetranitromethane

Trinitroaniline
Trinitroanisole
Trinitrobenzene
Trinitrochlorobenzene
2,4,6-trinitro-m-cresol
Trinitrotoluene
2,4,6-trinitroxylene
Zinc peroxide

Highly dangerous—gives off highly toxic fumes on heat, flame, shock

Carbon disulfide
Carbon monoxide
Carbon oxysulfide
Dibromoacetylene
Diethyl ether
Dimethyl ether
Ethyl nitrite
Hyponitrous acid
Mercury
Mercuric perchlorate
Methyl phosphine
Phosgene
Thionyl chloride-fluoride
Thiophosgene
Vinyl chloride
Vinyl ether
Vinylidene chloride

SPECIAL

Dangerous—when exposed to heat or flame may explode or is spontaneously flammable in air

Acetyl benzoyl peroxide
Acetylene
Acetylene chloride
Alkyl ethers <C_4
Allylene

(continued)

Aluminum chlorate
Ammonium chromate
Benzoyl peroxide, dry
Butadiene-1, 3
Chlorates
Dialkyl phosphines
Diazoacetic ester
Diazoamidobenzol
Diazobenzene chloride
Diethyl carbonate
Diisopropyl & higher-alkyl
  ethers
Ferrous perchlorate
Furan
Hydrazine, anhydrous
Hydrazoic acid
Hydrides, volatile
Hydrogen, cyanide (un-
  stabilized)
Hydrogen (low pressure)
Hydrogen peroxide
  (>35% water)
Magnesium peroxide
Mercurous azide
Methyl acetylene
Methyl lactate
Nickel hypophosphite
Nitriles ethyl
Nitrogen bromide
Inorganic salts of alkyl nitrates
Nitrosoguanidine
Nitrosomethyl urea (dry)
Ozone
Ozonides (solution)
Pentaborane
Perbenzoic acid
Perchlorates
Perchloric acid (10% or
  more water)
Performic acid
Peroxides (organic)
Phosphorus (white)

Phenylazoimide
Silicon hydride
Silver oxalate
Sodium chlorite
Trinitrobenzaldehyde

Dangerous—will react with
 water or steam to produce
 hydrogen toxic fumes or
 highly flammable gases

Acetone
Alkali cyanides, hydrides,
  sodium, & other metals
Aluminum borohydride,
  carbide, chloride, hydride,
  and nitride
Benzoyl chloride
Boron compounds
Carbonyls
Chlorine
Cyanogen bromide
Cyanogen chloride
Dialkyl carbamyl chlorides
Dialkyl cyanamide
Dialkyl aluminum hydrides
Diborane
Dibromoketone
Dichloromethyl chloro-
  formate
Diphosgene
Fuming nitric acid
Grignard's reagents
Hydrides (nonvolatile)
Hydrogen cyanide (stabilized)
Hydrogen fluoride
Lithium aluminum hydride
Magnesium metal
Nitric acid
Oleum
Phosphenyl chloride
Phosphides

(continued)

Phosphorus nitride, oxy-
halides, pentahalides &
trihalides
Radioisotopes, beta emitters
Sodium azide

CONVENTIONAL

*When heated to decomposition
gives off highly toxic fumes
or products that may be explosion hazards when exposed
to flame*

Acetic acid
Acetic anhydride
Acetoacetanilide
Acetone cyanohydrin
Acetyl chloride
Acrolein
Acrylonitrile
Alcohols
Alkaloids
Alkyl aryl acids, alcohols,
amines, esters, ethers $>C_3$,
halides, hydrocarbons,
ketones, mercaptans, &
sulfides
Alkyl dihalides
Alkyl nitrates
Allyl amine
Allyl cyanide
Allyl ether
Allyl halide
Amines
Aminoacetophenone
p-aminoazobenzene
p-aminophenol
2-amino pyridine
Amino pyrine
2-aminothiazole
Ammonia

Ammonium nitrate
Amyl nitrite
Aniline
Benzene sulfonyl chloride
Benzoyl peroxide (wet)
Bromine & iodine
N-bromoacetamide
Chlorobutanol
Chloroform
2-chloropyridine
Cresols
Cyanates
N, N-dialkylaminoethylamine
Dibutylphosphite
Dicyandiamide
Diethylamino ethanol
Diethyl phosphite
Diethyl sulfate
Diketene
Epichlorohydrin
Esters
Ethylene imine
Hydrazine hydrate
Hydrogen sulfide
Hydroxylamine salts
Inorganic Hg compounds
Iodates
Iodides
Ketones $>C_3$
Methyl acrylate
Methylene chloride
Nitriles
Nitrosomethyl urea (wet)
Petroleum ether
Piperidine
Propargyl bromide
Pyridine
Sodium alkoxide
Sodium azide
Sodium borohydride
Tetrabromoethane
Tetrachlorethane

(continued)

Moderately stable—when heated gives off acid fumes	Chlorophenyl carbamate
	Diethylene glycol
	Dimethyl formamide
Alcohol	Formic acid
Alkyl acids $>C_2$	Hydrocarbons
Alumina	Inorganic acids
Ammonia	Methyl diacetoacetate
Amyl alcohol	Phenyl cellosolve
Benzoic anhydride	Silica gel
Benzophenone	Tetradecane
Charcoal	Tetrahydrophthalic anhydride

Reprinted with permission from Safety Committee: Safety Handbook. Fairbanks, University of Alaska, 1977

Chemical Spills

Accidental spills are an unavoidable fact of laboratory work. They may be due to human error or faulty equipment. Spills are potentially dangerous, and steps must be taken to minimize the consequences to both personnel and property in serious spill cases. One such step is to establish an emergency spill-response person or team in each laboratory. Spill-response planning should include consideration of the types and amounts of chemicals and equipment used and the hazards associated with each one. Neutralizing agents (*e.g.,* sodium bicarbonate, sodium bisulfate) and absorbents (*e.g.,* vermiculite, sand) should be located strategically around the laboratory. If preferred, commercial kits are available that include everything required for all types of spill response. Protective apparel and spill-control and cleanup materials are essential throughout the laboratory.

Chemicals Spilled on the Skin

When a chemical is spilled on the skin, all of the contaminated clothing should be removed as quickly as possible and the area of skin should be flushed well and continuously for 15 minutes under a safety shower or in a sink, as appropriate. Wash the chemical off with soap or a mild detergent and water. Do *not* use neutralizing agents, creams, lotions, or salves on the skin. Obtain medical attention as soon as possible.

When a Spill Occurs

When a spill occurs, all persons in the immediate area should be notified and evacuated if necessary. If the material is flammable, all ignition and heat sources should be turned off. A respirator should be used, when necessary, to avoid breathing vapors during evacuation or cleanup. After it has been determined that there is proper ventilation and sufficient evaporation has occurred, the cleanup operation may proceed.

Commercial kits such as the Laboratory Spill Control Center from J. T. Baker Chemical Company include separate kits for the complete neutralizing and cleanup of concentrated acids, caustics, flammable solvents, mercury, cyanide, and hydrofluoric acid. These kits take the guesswork out of spill response and lessen the chances of worsening the effect. Commercial kits should be considered for all laboratories using chemicals.

Containment, Confinement, Dissipation, and Cleanup

Small liquid spills (<100 ml) can be readily absorbed and disposed of by the use of sand, paper towels, and neutralizer. Solid spills can be brushed onto a dustpan by a person using gloved hands and taking care to avoid reactive combinations of chemicals in the waste container. Either type of cleanup should be followed with soap-and-water mopping of the spill area and drying well. Acid-chloride spills require calcined absorbent products; alkali metals should be smothered with powdered graphite or commercial extinguisher and removed for further disposal.

Spilled mercury, which is extremely volatile and toxic, should be completely and immediately vacuumed up by a proper mercury-cleanup unit—not a domestic vacuum. Small droplets that are inaccessible to vacuuming may be converted to mercury sulfide with powdered sulfur or sodium-polysulfide solution. Do not place elemental mercury in laboratory drains.

Waste Disposal

Proper waste disposal is essential to a safe, clean laboratory and is a strict requirement of laws and regulations. Improper waste disposal puts not only laboratory workers, but also maintenance personnel and the surrounding community at risk. The laboratory supervisor must be well informed on local regulations and must set rules for the staff on what can or cannot be flushed down sinks or disposed of in solid waste containers (Table 3-11).

Each laboratory worker must keep hazardous and nonhazardous waste separated and all laboratories must have plainly marked containers to separate the waste generated. Unwanted solids should be discarded in a covered solids receptacle, and *only* waste paper should be put into the waste-paper container. Broken glassware must be discarded into a separate glassware container. Nonflammable water-soluble liquids may be flushed down the sink, but only small quantities of

Table 3-11. Chemicals Requiring Special Handling

CHEMICAL	COMMENTS	HANDLING AND DISPOSAL
Picric acid	High explosive; used in WW I military shells; extremely sensitive to shock	If chemical has dried out and become crystalline, try to open container GENTLY. Do not use force. Do not jolt container. If unable to open, dissolve substance in acetone or methyl hydrate, transport to a safe site, and detonate from a safe distance.
Diethyl ether	Watch for bulging of container; watch for crystals around top, or any signs of deterioration; forms explosive peroxides on deterioration	DO NOT ATTEMPT TO OPEN CONTAINER. Do not jolt or shake contents. Transport to safe area and open container remotely. Burn contents Highly explosive.
Barium peroxide	Highly explosive and unstable; sensitive to light, shock, and temperature change	Do not jolt. Maintain contents at room temperature. Remove to safe area and destroy remotely by detonation if possible.

(continued)

Table 3-11. Chemicals Requiring Special Handling (continued)

CHEMICAL	COMMENTS	HANDLING AND DISPOSAL
Other peroxides	Varying degrees of sensitivity	Handle cautiously, depending on type of peroxide. Destroy as above or by solution in water.
Phosphorus (red and yellow)	Very flammable and explosive if tightly contained	Maintain under water in original container. If contents dry out, do not attempt to open container.
Sodium and potassium metals	Very flammable in small quantities; very explosive in quantities over ½ oz., if in contact with air	Maintain under light oil. Destroy remotely in a safe area.
Carbon disulfide	Extremely poisonous; can be absorbed through the skin; causes severe liver toxicity; cumulative	Handle only with rubber gloves. Destroy remotely by burning. DO NOT BREATHE FUMES OR GASES GIVEN OFF BY BURNING.
Heavy metals (*e.g.*, mercury, lead, arsenic)	High toxicity; cumulative poison	Only satisfactory method of disposal is deep burial. Contact oil companies to dispose of materials in abandoned wells if you have a large quantity.
Halogens (*e.g.*, bromine, chlorine)	Extremely toxic; extremely corrosive	Have respiratory equipment at hand when disposing. Destroy remotely by chemical reaction.
Radioactive material		Observe usual precaution

Reprinted with permission from Fabian JT (ed): Chemistry safety. Monogr Calgary Board of Education, 1977

insolubles may be disposed of in this way. Flammables and insoluble liquids should be treated separately. Special instructions and methods must be given for waste mercury, sodium, alkali metals, and hydrides of alkali metals. Strong acids and bases should be diluted before being poured into the sink. Remember that laboratory sinks are often interconnected and stopped sinks or fugitive vapors can cause unplanned reactions if chemicals meet inadvertently. Containers that have held chemicals must be disposed of as chemical waste, not paper waste. When waste containers are small in size and they must be removed frequently, hazards in the laboratory are minimized.

Good Laboratory Practices for Clinical Chemistry

Chemical-Reagent Handling (Figs. 3-11, 3-12, 3-13)

- Limit quantities and concentrations of chemicals on hand to OSHA, NFPA, and local requirements.
- Clearly and permanently label all chemical containers to indicate the chemical contents and the hazards involved in their use. Reread all labels before using a chemical.
- Discard all unlabeled bottles.
- Fill a reagent bottle with only the material indicated by the label.
- Always flush the outsides of corrosive-chemical containers before and after use.
- Pour acid into water—never water into acid. (This helps to avoid splattering.)
- Do not lay stoppers down on any surface, because persons may accidentally come into contact with the wet surface.
- Keep all chemical containers tightly stoppered.
- Do not pour oil, grease, mercury, ether, or other solvents into laboratory sinks or drains because collected vapors present an explosion hazard.
- Dilute acids and alkalis before discarding them into sinks and follow this by flushing with large amounts of water.
- When handling toxic chemicals or flammable liquids or when a procedure may involve the production of toxic fumes, be sure that the process is performed in a well-ventilated area, preferably with a fume hood.
- Remember that the toxic effects of some fumes are cumulative

and that daily exposure to such fumes (*e.g.,* mercury) may lead to poisoning.

- Be careful when smelling chemicals. Never hold the container directly under the nose; hold it away and gently fan the vapors toward the nose.
- Use only the top of the lungs when smelling chemicals, filling the lungs first with clean air so that fumes can be expelled from the upper respiratory tract and nose.
- When holding flasks, beakers, or other glassware containing reagents to the light for examination, be sure to hold the vessel at a safe distance in order to avoid spilling the contents into the eyes or on your person.
- Fill reagent bottles to within one fourth of their capacity. This will permit the liquid adequate space for thermal expansion.

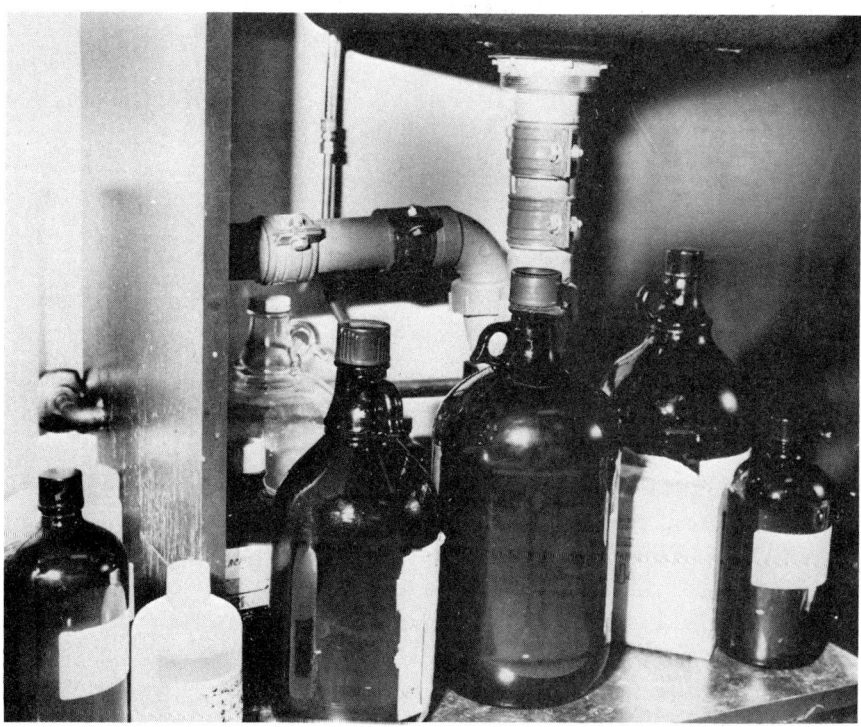

Fig. 3-11. Corrosive chemicals are better stored near the floor than on upper shelves.

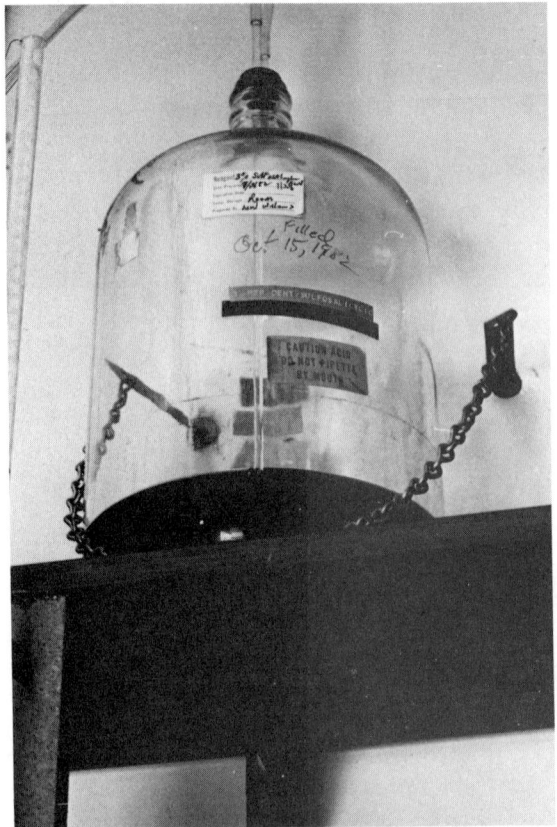

Fig. 3-12. If corrosives are dispensed from a shelf, they must be chained in place.

- Do not stopper bottles of alkaline solutions or solutions containing significant quantities of soluble salts with glass stoppers. Use clean, washed rubber stoppers.
- When heating a beaker of liquid on a hot plate, use a beaker cover to prevent spattering.
- Always wipe bench tops clean before and after use, because drops of acid or other corrosive chemicals may cause severe burns to others. Remove all spilled combustibles and volatiles immediately.
- If acids are spilled on the body, immediately rinse with copious amounts of water. Do not use neutralizing solutions in the eye or on the skin.
- Never taste any chemical.

- When pipetting chemicals, use a safety pipetting device.
- Open gas flames are not permitted in the vicinity of operations involving flammable liquids. Smoking is *not* allowed in the laboratory at all.
- Do not pour large volumes of volatile or flammable materials down the sink.
- Chemical disposal should take place in accordance with local regulations.
- Refrigeration will not prevent the formation of peroxides in ether.
- Purchase ether containing a peroxide inhibitor (water, iron, lead, or aluminum will *not* prevent peroxide formation in all ethers).
- Do not use alcohol to wash phenol off the skin. Alcohol only serves to spread the phenol—scrub instead with soap and water.

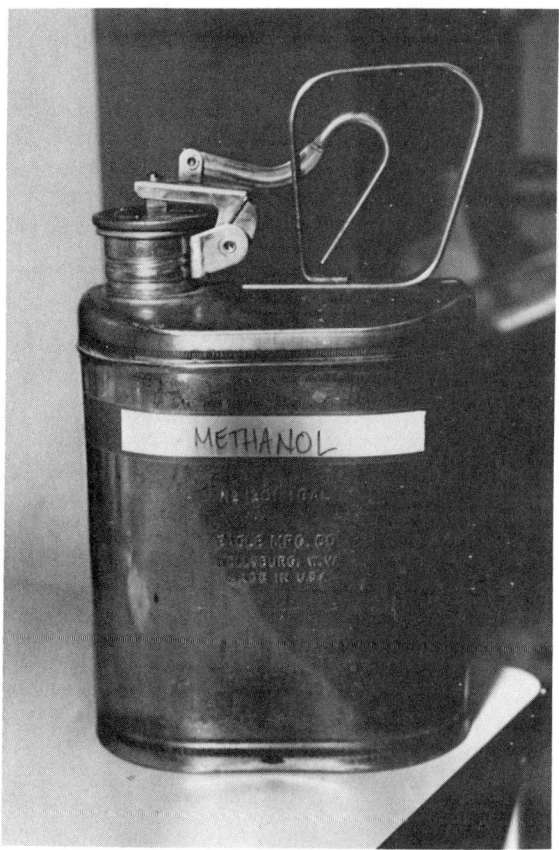

Fig. 3-13. One example of the many safety cans available for flammables.

- Carry beakers, reagent bottles, and flasks in a safety tray or with fingers around the body of the item.
- Treat all chemicals as potential hazards.
- Open operations with toxic solvents and evaporations of flammable, combustible, or toxic solvents must be carried out in a fume hood. Ovens must not be used for these evaporations.
- Clean spills immediately, using rags or an all-purpose absorbent. Dispose of the rags in a safety container that is emptied regularly.
- Centrifuge Class-I solvents only in explosion-proof refrigerators (see Classification of Flammable and Combustible Liquids, earlier in this chapter).
- When splashing, spraying, fire, or explosion may occur, adequate eye protection must be worn.
- Do not use more of a chemical than directed, and remove from the container only approximately what is needed. Never return excess of a chemical to its original container.
- Always add reagents slowly. Never "dump" them in. Pour concentrated solutions slowly into less concentrated solutions while stirring.
- Never look down the opening of a vessel unless it is empty.

Glassware Safety

Cuts, burns, and other accidents involving glassware represent a high percentage of laboratory accidents. Although most glassware accidents are not severe, careful adherence to established safety procedures and practices is necessary to minimize their frequency.

Glassware—General*

Damaged glassware is one of the most common sources of injuries in the laboratory. Chipped, cracked, or badly etched equipment or glassware with exposed sharp edges must be either repaired, fire polished, or discarded.

- Do not leave pipettes sticking out of bottles, flasks, or beakers

---

*Portions of this section are adapted with permission from Recommended Practice, Department of Environmental Health and Safety, University of Minnesota, Minneapolis, MN.

- Do not attempt to remove stoppers on glass tubing by forcing. If they are stuck, cut them off.
- Decontaminate glass exposed to specimens possibly containing hepatitis virus.
- Dispose of broken or discarded glass pieces in a specially marked and separate container. Disposal of broken glass along with paper and trash is an unnecessary hazard to the custodial staff.
- Heated glass containers should be handled with a heat-resistant glove.
- Glassware that is to be heated should be Pyrex or a similar heat-treated type.
- Fingers should never be used to pick up broken glass. A whisk broom and dustpan can be used for large pieces of glass. Use tongs to retrieve large pieces of glass in sinks and wet cotton held by tongs to retrieve chips and slivers.
- All glassware should be thoroughly cleaned after use.
- Laboratory glassware must never be used for eating or drinking.
- Glass objects that present breakage hazards should be wrapped for safety with plastic wire, wire screening, tape, or other special devices (*e.g.,* safety rings on graduated cylinders).
- Remember that heated glassware looks cool several seconds after heating but can still burn skin.
- Empty all glassware and rinse before setting aside for washing. Containers that have held toxic or corrosive chemicals should be made safe before washing.
- Guard against breaking the fragile neck of a volumetric flask by holding the stopper with thumb and forefinger and inserting stoppers with a gentle twisting motion.
- Store and use carboys and 5-gal bottles in the crates provided. Avoid handling large unprotected glass containers filled with liquid. Remember that large bottles (Pyrex included) are susceptible to thermal shock.
- The liquid level in containers provided with a positive closure should leave a 10% air space.
- Vessels with positive closures should not normally be placed in a steam bath or subjected to direct heat.
- Beakers, flasks, and bottles should be protected by asbestos-centered gauze when heating by direct flame.
- Beakers or flasks of over 1 liter must not be heated by flames or placed into direct contact with a hot plate.

- Avoid heating of soft glass vessels by any means.
- Flasks should always be supported at the bottom with a neck clamp.
- Large flasks and beakers should be supported by a tripod, not by ring clamps.
- Ground-glass connections should be lubricated before assembly and disassembled immediately after use.
- Frozen ground-glass joints should not be forced open.
- Use a stopcock puller to remove frozen stopcocks or ground-glass stoppers. The use of heat is not recommended and must never be used if the content is unknown or is affected by heat.
- Store glassware well back on the shelf, placing large heavy pieces on lower shelves.
- Glassware to be subjected to pressure or vacuum shall be Pyrex glass, heavy-walled if the vessel has a flat bottom; and carefully inspected for flaws before use.

Glassware Cleaning

Acid-type glassware cleaners combine the hazards of a strong oxidizing agent and a corrosive acid. Mixing chemicals with the cleaner releases considerable heat, which may break or damage plastic containers. Follow these procedures when using glassware cleaners:

- Use a face shield or splashproof safety goggles to protect eyes.
- Use long rubber gloves and aprons to protect the body.
- Use tongs or special perforated containers for handling objects that have been immersed in the cleaning solution.
- Immediately clean up spills on the skin, floors, and so on.
- Wash hands well after using cleaning solution.
- Remember when preparing cleaning solution that the heat of reaction can destroy the container.
- Store cleaning solutions separately from combustibles and organic or other oxidizable chemicals.
- Use the cleaning solution in a deep sink or container.

Cutting Glass Tubing

- Lay the tubing on a flat surface and hold it firmly in place with the hand at the approximate location where the break is to be made.

- At the location where the cut is desired, produce a deep scratch by drawing the edge of a triangular file firmly across the tube.
- If gloves are not available, use a cloth to cover the tube in the area in which the break is to be made.
- Grasp the covered tube with both hands so that the scratch is on the outer side, the fingers circling the tube, and the thumbs meeting on the opposite side behind the scratch.
- Sharp edges must be fire polished.
- Lubricant (glycerine, for example) should be used when inserting glass tubing into rubber stoppers and flexible tubing. Never use excessive force. Protect hands and fingers with gloves or towels.
- To avoid breakage, slit flexible tubing and rubber stoppers before removing them from glass.

Glassware Under Stress

- Systems operating at high pressure or vacuum must be shielded or guarded. Effective protection may be screen or metal containers, a nonfracturing overwrap of plastic or metal, glass-fiber taping, or a plastic dip coating.
- Safety devices, such as positive pressure relief valves or a slit in a rubber tubing connection, should be incorporated into the system so that excessive pressure can be relieved.
- Glass columns containing ion-exchange beads must be wrapped with tape or otherwise protected if the beads can expand and fracture the glass.

Drying With Air

- Compressed air pressure from the line must not exceed 30 psi.
- The air line should be opened slowly and any foreign matter blown out before it is connected to any glass system.
- Air must be introduced into the smallest opening of glassware to avoid excessive pressure buildup.
- Never hold your face or body over glassware while it is being air dried or point the drying article at any other person.

4

Blood Bank, Serology, and Radioimmunoassay

THE BLOOD BANK AND SEROLOGY LABORATORY

When the blood bank or immunohematology laboratory is called a high-risk laboratory, the risk referred to is to the patient—not to the technical staff. The hazards to the employee in this laboratory are among the easiest to control of those in the various clinical laboratory departments. In this chapter, however, the concern *is* with the technician and with those hazards, however subtle, that may be encountered in serologic or blood-banking procedures.

Compared with other laboratories, such as the chemistry laboratory, the blood bank and serology laboratory are relatively benign places to work; there are few chemical hazards, no pressurized gases, and little or no sophisticated electronic equipment. However, the hazard of contracting infectious hepatitis, especially from the sera of posttransfusion patients, is extremely high. In addition, other infectious agents may be encountered in the sera. For this reason, the discussion of hepatitis in Chapter 5 should be carefully read and understood by blood bankers. This chapter addresses hepatitis only in conjunction with the hepatitis-associated antigen (HAA) test and other blood-banking and serologic procedures in which hepatitis precautions are especially important. All reagents and sera of human origin in the blood bank and in all serology laboratories must, of course, be treated as potential sources of hepatitis and handled accordingly.

Stop for a moment and watch a blood bank at work. The kinds and amounts of aerosol production in blood-banking procedures will probably surprise you. Remember that not only puncture wounds transmit hepatitis and infectious disease. Do not be lulled into a false sense of security by a clean, well-run blood bank or serology laboratory with its few reagents and seemingly unlimited antigens and antibodies.

Although cautious handling of serum and avoidance of aerosol production should afford the blood-bank technician a low-risk job, neat, careful work habits and a clean workspace are also essential. A safety-conscious, well-organized blood bank or serology laboratory where there is concern for keeping a healthy and accident-free staff is also of benefit to the patient, the ultimate beneficiary of a well-run laboratory. Remember that in only the blood bank does the product of laboratory procedures go directly into the patient—via transfusions. These same transfusions produce the hepatitis risk to the blood-bank and serology staff.

This chapter begins with some general rules of good laboratory practice for the blood-bank and serology laboratory. This is followed by a section on quality control and diagnostic sera, which are additional hepatitis hazards, and a short discussion on performing various HAA tests safely. The chapter continues with the proper safety methods for fluorescence microscopy and a brief statement on other hazards encountered in the blood bank and serology laboratory and concludes with a section on the radioimmunoassay laboratory.

Good Laboratory Practices for the Blood Bank and Serology Laboratory

- Proper laboratory attire should be worn at all times (laboratory coats, closed-toe shoes, etc.).
- No smoking, drinking, or eating is allowed in the laboratory, nor is storage of food permitted in blood-bank refrigerators (Fig. 4-1).

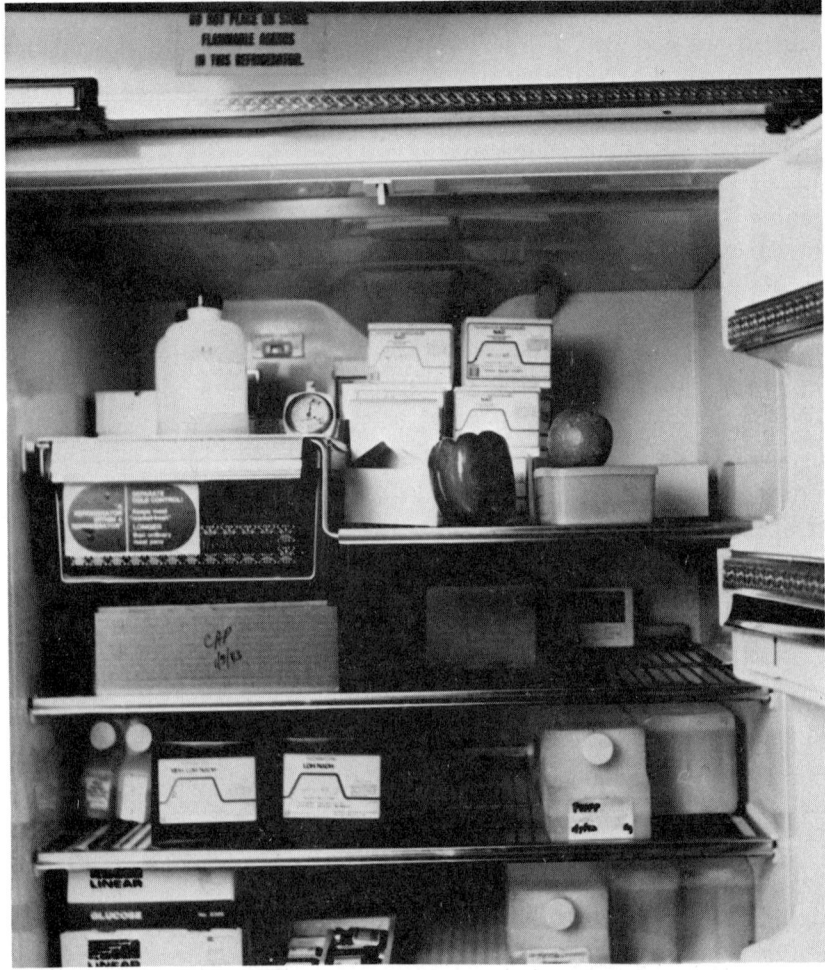

Fig. 4-1. Food may not be placed in the laboratory refrigerator or consumed in the laboratory. This represents a safety violation.

- Beware of dumping reagents that contain sodium azide (*e.g.,* blood-bank reagents) into sinks.
- If azide-containing reagents must be used, flush the sink well or put azide waste into bags and dispose of them with solid waste.
- Use disposables wherever possible, including tubes, mixing sticks, and so on.
- A vast amount of aerosols is created in the mixing, decanting,

squirting, and centrifuging for crossmatching and serologies, and extra care must be exercised in these procedures.

- Properly discard all biohazardous samples and contaminated materials in the proper biohazard bags, and the paper waste in separate waste containers.
- All serum specimens should be discarded according to the individual laboratory rules after testing is finished. This usually includes autoclaving of known hepatitis-containing sera.
- Clip or recover all needles or place them in impervious containers as laboratory policy dictates.
- All glass and broken glass should be discarded so that the housekeeping and maintenance staff will not accidentally be punctured. Bags should be labeled to identify the contents as BROKEN GLASS.
- Blood-bank reagents and all test and control reagents should be shown to be hepatitis B surface antigen (HB_sAg) negative and labeled *HAA negative*. It should be remembered that non-A, non-B hepatitis may still be transmitted even when the HAA test is negative. Additionally, some HAA positives may not be picked up in HAA testing.
- Wash hands often because handwashing physically removes infectious material and soap denatures microbial proteins.
- Do not use pooled human sera for any procedures.
- After spills and at the end of the work shift, use diluted Clorox solution to clean bench tops. Wear gloves while cleaning with Clorox solution.
- Do not use phenol and Clorox together because chlorine gas may be released.
- Always use a bulb to reconstitute or mix; never mouth pipette (Fig. 4-2).
- Do not leave pipettes sticking out of tubes or reagent bottles.
- When centrifuging (serofuging), always use the safety latch and allow the acrosol to settle before opening if tubes have shattered.
- Sera from known hepatitis patients should be well wrapped and should be autoclaved or incinerated before final disposal. While you are performing laboratory procedures, handle sera from known hepatitis patients carefully and preferably with gloves.
- A cluttered work area with samples, equipment, cords, reagents, and so on scattered about can lead to accidents, spills, or falls. A tidy work area will considerably cut down on accidents.

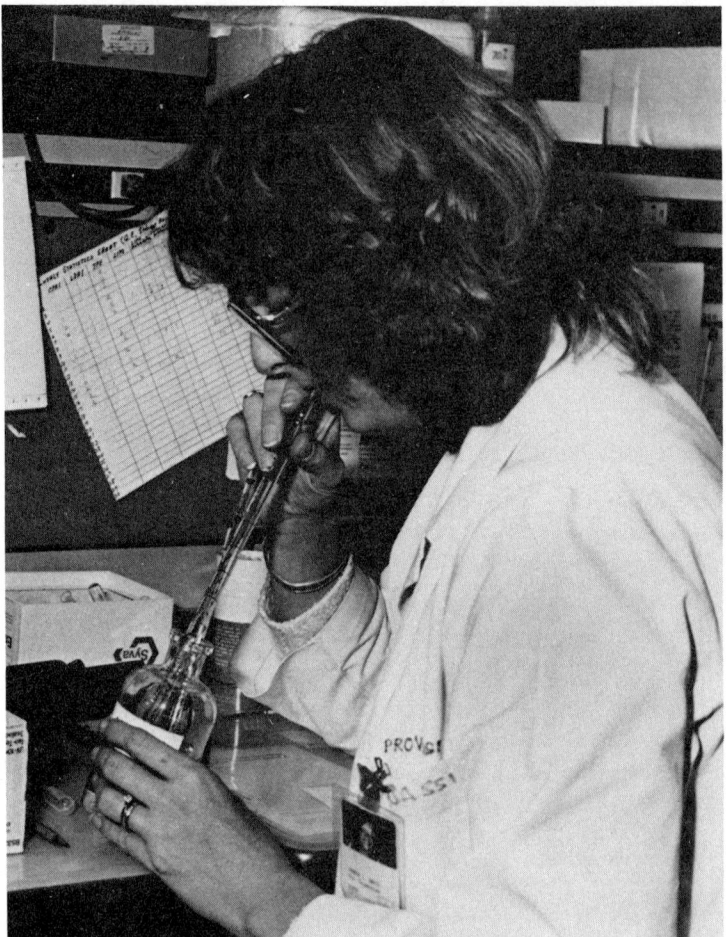

Fig. 4-2. Mouth pipetting is *not* allowed in the laboratory, even when a substance appears innocuous. The risks of infection and toxicity are too great to overlook.

Control and Diagnostic Sera—Another Hepatitis Hazard

In 1973, a serious but previously unrecognized laboratory hazard was identified—hepatitis B antigen positive typing and control sera.* In tests of 135 samples by a radioimmunoassay technique; 33.3% contained

*Weill CV et al: A previously unrecognized laboratory hazard: Hepatitis B antigen-positive control and diagnostic sera. Am J Clin Pathol 59:681–687, 1973

demonstrable HB$_s$Ag (Table 4-1). It was concluded that both commercial and laboratory-made typing sera and serum controls present a serious serum-hepatitis hazard to all laboratory workers; that stringent, strictly enforced safety precautions should be instituted in all clinical laboratories to minimize exposure to the agent of serum hepatitis; and that manufacture of such sera should minimize the potential health hazard of these products.

Since this and other findings were published, reagent manufacturing often includes HAA testing and most reagents are now labeled HAA negative. However, technicians should bear in mind that HAA testing cannot detect all levels of HAA and not all products are tested (*e.g.,*

Table 4-1. Control and Diagnostic Sera Positive for Hepatitis B Antigen

REAGENTS TESTED BY TYPE	NUMBER TESTED	NUMBER POSITIVE	% POSITIVE
Chemistry	46	28	61
Control sera			
Enzyme controls			
Automated control sera			
Pooled plasma			
Quality-control survey sera			
Hematology	25	10	40
Coagulation controls			
Coagulation reagents			
Blood-grouping reagents			
Immunohematology reagents			
Serology	17	4	24
Test control serum			
Test reagent serum			
Test controls and reagents			
Microbiology	47	3	6
Bacteriologic typing sera			
Febrile agglutination reagents			
Total	135	45	33.3

(Adapted from Weill CV et al: A previously unrecognized laboratory hazard: Hepatitis B antigen-positive control and diagnostic sera. Am J Clin Pathol 59:681–687, 1973)

those made in the laboratory). All products made from pooled human plasma or serum should be treated as potential hepatitis sources, and whenever possible only those labeled HAA negative should be used.

Performing the HAA Test Safely

Despite the lack of definitive identification of the hepatitis virus in laboratory culture, it has been shown that hepatitis disease can be transmitted in the positive controls and serum samples used in HAA testing. Some suggestions follow on additional precautions to be used in various types of HAA procedures. Currently, the procedure of choice for HAA is the radioimmunoassay, but other tests are still used in some laboratories and will be discussed. Awareness of safe working methods is important in itself.

HAA General Precautions

Always pipette with a rubber bulb or other safety device and keep the pipette plugged with cotton to avoid bulb contamination. Even noninfectious reagents may not be pipetted by mouth. Perform work over plastic-backed paper and do not empty test vessels prior to decontamination because of aerosol creation. Wear gloves whenever necessary and possible and remember not to contaminate other items with a contaminated glove.

Immunodiffusion Techniques

When performing immunodiffusion techniques, the flat glass slide becomes contaminated in processing of this test and spreads moisture to the slide holder. This creates a hazard during the reading of reactions. Using a Petri dish to hold the slides or gel while performing the test minimizes hazard. Staining of the slides or gel is not recommended because of the risk of contamination during rinsing and the small (if any) degree of differentiation staining will provide. Rather than stain, use a black background against oblique light to read the reactions. Forceps used in handling slides should be autoclaved.

Immunoelectroosmophoresis

Immunoelectroosmophoresis (IEOP) procedures present the same problems that immunodiffusion does but additionally wicks, buffer, and the chamber may become contaminated as well. Wear gloves for placing plates into the chamber, adjusting wicks, and removing plates after completion. Autoclave all test parts. Aspirate buffer from the chamber into a closed flask and autoclave. Again, staining is not recommended. The electrical hazard in this test is also a serious hazard. The IEOP test should be performed only by technicians who are well trained in its safety risks and proper operation. Proper grounding and enclosure of electrophoresis equipment is essential.

Complement Fixation Tests, Microtiter Method

For complement fixation tests, use disposable plastic plates and autoclave all blotters. Decontaminate microdiluters by boiling. Diluent and rinse-water containers are autoclaved when full. Test cups should be covered with nonabsorbent cardboard and wrapped in plastic film. Do not seal them with masking tape. After the incubation period for complement fixation, lay back the plastic film, remove the cardboard to a discard pan, add red blood cells to the plate, tape-seal to contain the contents, and cover everything with plastic film. These precautions minimize spills, aerosols, and contamination.

Fluorescence Microscopy

Fluorescent microscopes require certain safety precautions during use and even more so during alignment because of their explosion potential and eye hazard. A fluorescent microscope contains an ultraviolet light source, which may, unfiltered, cause retinal burns. It also has a high-pressure mercury bulb, which may implode.

These safety practices will serve to remind the laboratory worker of the potential problems encountered in fluorescent microscopy:

- Take care at all times during alignment or changing mercury-pressure lamp to avoid any direct contact with the ultraviolet light.

- The ultraviolet light should *always* be shielded and filtered.
- During alignment, make sure the proper filter is in place before viewing the specimen.
- When changing the mercury-pressure lamp or when the lamp housing is open, be sure that the power cord is unplugged. This is a high-voltage precaution as well as a safety practice due to the dangers of mercury-bulb implosions. It is advisable to wear safety goggles or a face shield when changing the lamp.
- When a unit is not in use from one day to the next, unplug the transformer from the wall outlet to prolong the life of the transformer.
- If the lamp has been in operation, do not open the housing until it has sufficiently cooled because of the danger of implosion.
- Routine maintenance and inspection should be performed on these microscopes as needed, but annually at a minimum.
- To dispose of mercury lamps, arrange to return them to the vendor or dispose of them as a hazardous substance.
- Fluorescent microscopes and all electrical equipment should be properly grounded.

Other Blood-Bank or Serologic Procedures in Which Hazards May Be Encountered

There are other blood-bank or serologic procedures in which hazards may be encountered. Among them are the following:

- Enzyme methods for crossmatching and antibody screening. These use enzymes such as papain, ficin, bromelin, and trypsin. Some strong individual reactions have been seen with dry ficin powder and wearing a mask is a good idea when reconstituting enzymes.
- Ether elution methods. These use diethyl ether. Extreme care should be exercised because ether can explode.
- Use of 2-mercaptoethanol to differentiate IgM from IgG. It has a very foul smell even when diluted and should be handled cautiously.
- Use of typing sera, which contains sodium azide as a preservative. Do not flush any reagents containing sodium azide into the sink undiluted.

- Use of noisy equipment. Noise in any laboratory may be a problem but in a relatively quiet laboratory like the blood bank, the constant sound of refrigerator compressors and serofuging may be an irritant and should be baffled whenever possible.
- Immunoelectrophoresis techniques. These combine electrophoretic separation of substances of different electric charges with separation by double diffusion in agar gel. Four volts to six volts per centimeter of direct current are used and create a substantial electrical hazard. Proper grounding of equipment and training of technicians are essential to avoid shock or burns.
- Use of hazardous chemicals. Mercury derivatives may be used in serology reagents as a preservative. Acetone and other flammables may also be used in the blood bank or serology laboratory. Proper techniques for these hazardous chemicals must be employed.
- Handling of human sera. Be aware that infectious agents other than hepatitis (*e.g., Treponema,* fungi, meningococcus) may be found in human sera and handle them accordingly.
- Serologic procedures with inactivated antigens. These can be performed on the open workbench, but residual infectivity may be a potential problem with some procedures. Disinfectants should be used in the water if water baths are used to inactivate, incubate, or test biohazardous materials.

THE RADIOIMMUNOASSAY LABORATORY

Although the radioimmunoassay (RIA) laboratory shares many of the potential hazards of the other clinical laboratories (*e.g.,* hepatitis potential, flammable chemicals), it also requires a unique set of precautions owing to the presence of very low levels of radiation. Because it has no odor and cannot be seen, tasted, or felt, radiation is apt to be treated as being of little consequence. The precautions to be used in an RIA laboratory are not indicative of significant hazard, but reflect routine good laboratory practice for handling radioactive material (Fig. 4-3).

A brief statement or two on radiation will provide an introduction for the discussion of safety techniques in the RIA laboratory. Radiation, defined as the *propagation of energy through space or matter,* can be either electromagnetic (*e.g.,* gamma rays) or particulate (*e.g.,* alpha

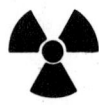 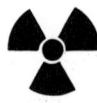

REMINDER OF GOOD RADIOISOTOPE LABORATORY SAFETY PRACTICES

1. Never pipette by mouth.

2. No smoking or eating permitted in the work area.

3. Gloves and laboratory coat are required when using radioactive materials.

4. Prescribed personnel monitors must be worn.

5. Hands, shoes and clothing should be frequently monitored.

6. Work with radioactive materials in an approved hood or glove box, unless the safety of working on an open bench can be demonstrated.

7. Radioisotope work should be conducted in an impervious tray or pan, lined with absorbent paper.

8. Utilize shielding and distance whenever possible.

9. Dispose of liquid and solid radioactive waste in the approved containers provided.

10. Refrigerators containing radioactive material shall not be used for storing food.

11. Monitor radioisotope work areas at least once daily for contamination and make notation of this survey in laboratory records.

12. Thoroughly wash hands after manipulating radioactive material, especially before eating or smoking, and on completion of work.

13. Maintain records of receipt, use, transfer and disposal of radioactive materials.

14. Report accidental inhalation, ingestion, injury or spills to your supervisor and the Radiation Safety Officer or appropriate official.

15. Review pertinent safety practices frequently, especially before using a new radioisotope.

If you have any questions or need assistance, contact the Radiation Safety Office before work begins.

Fig. 4-3. This notice should be posted in a conspicuous place in a laboratory using radioisotopes.

rays, beta rays, neutrons). The biological hazard of either type of ionizing radiation is damage to the DNA in the cell nucleus from the transfer of this energy. Each type of radiation has its own particular hazards and precautions. With very high radiation doses, not found in the RIA laboratory, this damage can result in cell death, cancer, or mutation. Doses such as these are *not* found in a diagnostic laboratory.

Obviously, radiation may be harmful. Control of exposure is based on the conservative assumption that *any* exposure involves some risk. However, current permissible occupational exposures are so low that no clinical effects have been shown at these levels.

Radiation experts have set the standards for permissible low-level exposures and continue to reassess them based on the assumption that some, as yet undetectable, effects may occur at levels approaching zero dose (Table 4-2). However, because of natural background radiation, a zero-dose level is not an achievable standard.

In handling radioactive materials, such as in RIA kits or nuclear-medicine procedures, care must be taken to avoid both external and internal contamination. Internal contamination, which is radioactivity

Table 4-2. Typical Radiation Exposure Limits

NATIONAL INSTITUTES OF HEALTH EMPLOYEE EXPOSURE LIMITS	ALLOWABLE EXPOSURE (mrem/yr)*
National Institutes of Health x-ray technician or nuclear-medicine worker	5000
National Institutes of Health fer-tile-age women employee	3000 (at rate of 250 mrem/mo)
General public—nonradiation workers	500
National Institutes of Health worker under 18 years old	500

*Millirem (mrec [1/1000 rem]) is a radiation dose equivalent taking into account biological effects of different types of ionizing radiation. The average person in the United States accumulates a dose of 1 rem/12 yr from natural sources.
From the United States Department of Health, Education and Welfare. NIH Radiation Safety Guide (NIH 79-18) 1979.

inside the body, would result from accidental inhalation, ingestion, skin absorption, or laceration. External exposure may result from handling source vials or spills. The severity of the effect depends on the half-life of the radioactive source, the type of radiation emitted, the penetrating power, the part of the body exposed, and the duration of exposure. In cases in which the radioactive material is taken into the body, as in accidental ingestion, continuous and damaging irradiation of cells and tissues may occur. An alpha particle cannot penetrate the skin, so it is harmless as an external danger; however, it does produce a different hazard internally, where it can be absorbed by bone and organs. Care must be taken to prevent this occurrence.

Radioisotopes (also called radionuclides) used in RIA are the radioactive forms of the elements. They behave chemically as do the nonradioactive stable forms. The RIA procedures use such low levels of radioactivity, however, that special radiation procedures and personnel monitoring often are not legally required. In those hospitals where RIA is part of nuclear medicine (the "hot laboratory"), RIA is regulated under the strict Nuclear Regulatory Commission (NRC) nuclear-medicine guidelines. The concern for radiation protection expressed here reflects the possibility that RIA may be part of the nuclear medicine laboratory and that working with RIA always requires a prudent approach. When proper safety guidelines are followed, workers in RIA laboratories will receive radiation exposures not detectably different from background levels.

License to Perform Tests and Employee Training

The type of license under which radioisotopes are obtained depends on the scope and size of the nuclear-medicine practice or the clinical *in vitro* tests performed. Under an NRC specific license, each hospital must have a radiation safety officer who is responsible for meeting the legal safety requirements for personnel surveillance and for monitoring, proper disposal, and proper handling of shipments of radioactive materials. The radiation safety officer must also keep inventories, provide advice, and continually evaluate use and hazards of radiation in the hospital. Training sessions for all personnel handling radioactive material are required annually, and topics covered should include health-protection problems, proper storage, transfer, and use of radioactive materials, and explanation of the presence and potential hazards of radionuclides found in the employees' work area. Wearing of film badges or thermoluminescent dosimeters by workers performing only *in vitro* RIA tests, however, is more a legal precaution than a safety concern.

Personnel are entitled to see their own exposure records and the hospital's or physicians' licenses. Additionally, the relevant NRC or OSHA rules and regulations should be conspicuously posted.

Pregnancy and the Radioimmunoassay Laboratory

The embryo and fetus are much more susceptible to the effects of radiation than is an adult. Thus women who are, or may be, pregnant must make a decision about continuing to work with radioactivity. Although this is not a problem in the average RIA laboratory, it may be a concern when RIA is part of nuclear medicine. Often, a woman's work in the hot laboratory is curtailed or eliminated until her pregnancy is over. Before making a decision to continue working in nuclear medicine, it is important for the pregnant medical technologist to discuss with her obstetrician and radiation safety officer her work options and the fetal risks involved.

Working With Isotopes

The average RIA procedures use ^{125}I, a gamma emitter, as the tracer radioactive component, although several other isotopes such as ^{3}H and ^{57}Co, ^{58}Co, and ^{59}Co are still found in some tests. Only one reagent per test is radioactive. Remember that other chemicals (flammables, corrosives, etc.) are also found in the RIA laboratory in controlled amounts and precautions should always be used as appropriate for these chemicals as well.

Isotopes are chosen for their chemical compatibility with the test procedure and their safety and detection qualities. Ease of detection at these low levels is a significant reason for choosing ^{125}I for RIA kits. ^{125}I also has a desirable half-life—60 days. This means it need not be used immediately and will decay to a very low level in a reasonable amount of time. An RIA kit has only 5 μCi of radioactivity per kit. A total of 200

μCi of radioactivity may be on hand at any one time under the provisions of the general license.

No matter what the level of radiation, radiation protection to the worker is increased by adequate shielding, greater distance from the tracer, and a limit to the amount of time spent with the radioactive material. Workers should open vials under a hood or at a distance, cover tubes with caps provided, and take care when adding labeled materials to test tubes. RIA kits are adequately shielded by thin lead foil.

Glassware and equipment used in the RIA laboratory should not be used in other laboratories. Additionally, when equipment malfunctions, repairs should not be made by unsupervised service personnel or sent to the shop before thorough decontamination has been performed.

Storage, Labeling, and Signs

All radioactive material should be appropriately shielded and stored in unbreakable containers. If the area where the material is stored is not itself restricted or locked, the refrigerator or freezer containing the material must be locked. A proper label should appear on each container of radioactive material, including materials made up in the laboratory. Signs indicating the presence of radioactive materials should be placed in the radionuclide storage area. Storage areas should be locked whenever laboratory personnel are not in attendance. RIA testing should be performed separately from nuclear-medicine and other chemical procedures. The radiation symbol should be displayed on the door, refrigerator, and hood, alerting personnel to the presence of radioactive material therein (Figs. 4-4 and 4-5).

Waste Disposal

Under guidelines governing users of the NRC general license, effluents from RIA *in vitro* tests may be flushed into the sink and diluted with large amounts of water. The amount of such disposal should not exceed 20 μCi per day. Unused isotopes may be allowed to decay in storage or returned to the supplier. Disposable paper and waste may safely be discarded with routine trash, but only after all radioactive labels are removed. If biohazards are present, autoclave RIA materials

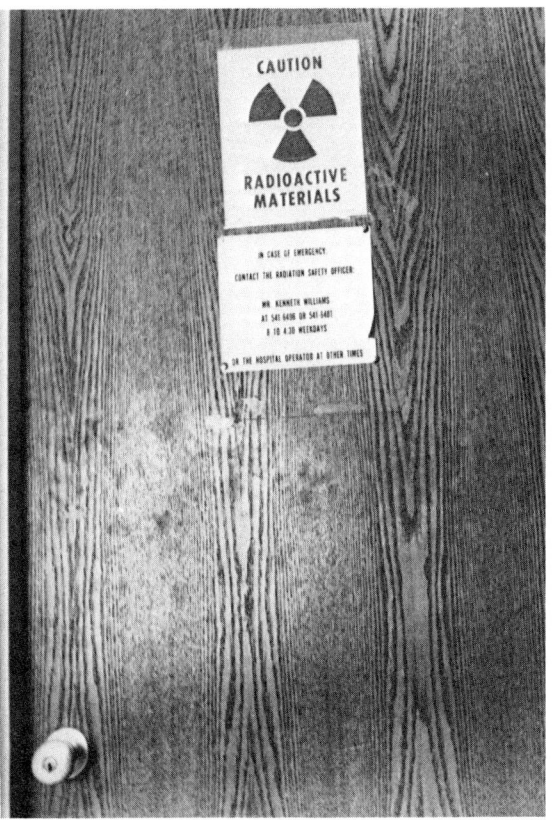

Fig. 4-4. The RIA laboratory should be separate and locked. The radioactive-materials sign must be prominently displayed on the door.

before disposal into trash or a sewer. Local jurisdictions may impose their own special disposal requirements, despite the very low levels of radioactivity involved.

RIA Shipments: Handling, Accountability, and Disposition

RIA *in vitro* diagnostics are of such low levels that special radiation-packaging procedures and labels are often not necessary or required. Radiation labels may not even appear externally on packages arriving at the laboratory. However, as with all radiation sources, damaged RIA packages should be handled carefully, monitored for

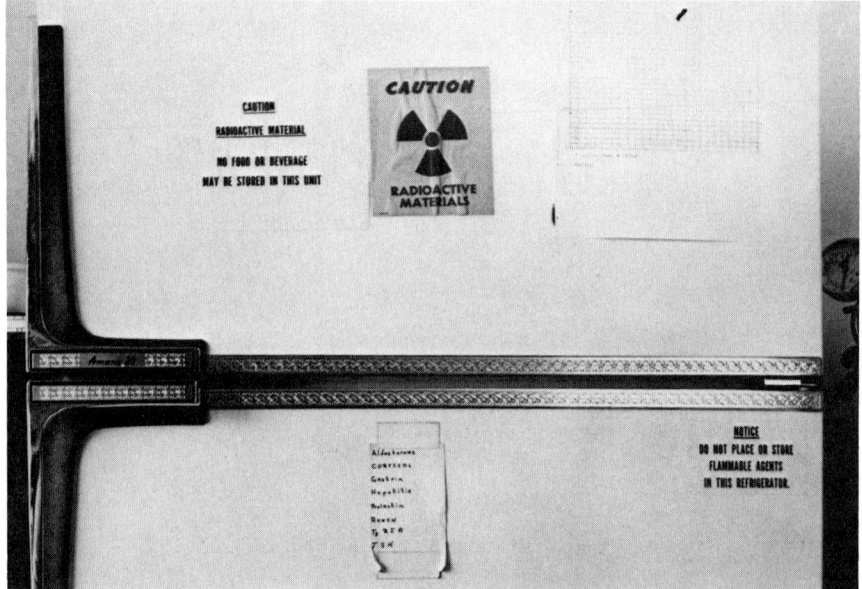

Fig. 4-5. Refrigerators containing radioactive materials must be so labeled and used for nothing else. If the laboratory itself is not locked, the refrigerator must be.

contamination, and opened with gloves. If the contents are disturbed or appear broken, they should be placed in an appropriate container to prevent further leakage. Areas in which a package has been leaking should also be surveyed for contamination. All shipments containing radioactive material must be logged in and a record must be kept of the material's ultimate disposition, be it used, discarded, or even spilled (Fig. 4-6).

Measurement Devices for Personnel and Area Monitoring

To ensure that protection against radiation is adequate and that there is adherence to safety rules and regulations, measurement devices are used to detect and measure radiation and provide a permanent record of worker exposure. These records should also be kept on file in the health unit for each employee so monitored. Personnel or laboratory contamination *must* be reported to the radiation safety officer.

Examples of measurement devices include the following:

ISOTOPE RECEIPT, UTILIZATION AND DISPOSAL RECORD

INSTRUCTIONS:
Fill out one form for each shipment received and keep on file in your laboratory.

NAME OF INVESTIGATOR

	BUILDING	ROOM NO.	DATE
ISOTOPE	ACTIVITY	CHEMICAL FORM	SPECIFIC ACTIVITY	SUPPLIER

ENTER BELOW WHEN ANY MATERIAL IS USED OR PLACED IN RADIOACTIVE WASTE CONTAINERS. YOU ARE REMINDED THAT THE NIH RADIATION SAFETY REGULATIONS DO NOT PERMIT ANY RADIOACTIVE RELEASES TO THE SEWER.

DATE OF USE	AMOUNT USED		DATE OF DISPOSAL	ACTIVITY DISPOSED	MANNER OF DISPOSAL (Liquid, solid, or animal carcasses)
	ACTIVITY	VOLUME			

RELEASES TO HOOD

DATE	ACTIVITY	DATE	ACTIVITY

COMMENTS:

Additional comments on back of form ☐

CDC 3.1116
3-80

Fig. 4-6. Radioactive-material disposal record.

- *Film badge*—photographic film that darkens upon exposure to radiation; the degree of darkening is correlated to degree of exposure. These are ideally worn for no longer than 1 month.
- *Pocket dosimeter*—electrically charged quartz fiber that gets discharged by radiation and moves across a scale visible through a lens. This provides a cumulative reading of exposure.
- *Thermoluminescent dosimeter (TLD)*—worn on a badge (or as a ring to check extremity exposure); small chips of lithium fluoride. A readout meter reads total dose and returns the dosimeter to zero. It can be worn longer than 1 month if exposure is low. To reflect exposure to personnel, dosimeters must be worn. For obvious reasons, they must not be stored or left near radioactive materials when not on the worker.
- *Detectors*—electronic instruments that read and record the ionizing radiation levels: Geiger counter, proportional counter, ionization chamber, scintillation counter. Detectors must be appropriate to type of radiation.
- *Routine monitoring*—will detect radioactive contamination and allow evaluation of shielding. Laboratory areas, such as RIA, that do not use much radioactive material should be surveyed monthly using a survey meter and a series of smear (or swipe) tests, although the workbench may be monitored daily. A permanent record should be kept of *all* survey results including negative results and should include drawings of the area, names of personnel, corrective action, and so on (Figs. 4-7). In addition to routine monitoring by the hospital, there may be monitoring by organizations such as the NRC for radiation when these organizations perform inspection visits. Halls and floors are also monitored to ensure that contamination has not spread.

Spill Cleanup: Personnel and Work Areas

Absorbent padding with a plastic backing should be used to cover work surfaces. In the event of spills or in normal use, these can be discarded in normal trash. If spills occur, use soap and water or commercial decontaminating agents such as Radiac Wash or Versene on the area until acceptable radiation levels are reached. Try to isolate the spill area and keep water volume as low as possible. When spills occur that affect personnel, remove the contaminated clothing. If a cut

RADIATION SURVEY REPORT

DEPARTMENT OF HEALTH, EDUCATION, AND WELFARE
PUBLIC HEALTH SERVICE
CENTER FOR DISEASE CONTROL
ATLANTA, GEORGIA 30333

EXAMPLE

| Authorized Investigator | Telephone ## |
| Surveyor | Telephone ## |

BUILDING SUFFIX   FLOOR   WING

Radionuclides used in this location:

MONTH   DAY   YEAR   AUTHORIZED USER NUMBER

COUNTING EQUIPMENT

L.S.C. __ EFF _____ %

GAMMA __ EFF _____ %

Area Diagram and Sampling Sites

SMEAR SURVEY RESULTS

Location	DPM	NUCLIDE	Location	DPM	NUCLIDE
1			6		
2			7		
3			8		
4			9		
5			10		

COMPLIANCE ITEMS

Room and Storage Posted ☐   Containers & Equipment Labeled ☐   Survey Records Adequate ☐

Inventory, Disposal Records Adequate ☐   Personnel Monitoring ☐   Bioassay/Whole Body Count ☐

Pipetting Devices ☐   Food, Drink, or Smoking ☐   Gloves, Lab Coats ☐

Absorbent Paper, Trays ☐   Waste Handling Practices ☐   Shielding ☐

Hoods and Ventilation ☐   Personnel Training ☐   Other. ☐

Survey Instruments ☐

ADDITIONAL INFORMATION, REMARKS

CDC 3.1114 2-80

Fig. 4-7. Sample format for radiation monitoring.

occurs, encourage bleeding to force out foreign material. When a corrosive chemical is being used, also follow procedures for chemical decontamination. Use soap and water or a designated commercial decontaminant for skin contamination, taking extreme care not to abrade the skin or open a portal of entry.

If other hazards are part of an accident (biological, chemical, or flammable hazards), do not forget appropriate cautions and cleanup for these hazards as well, dealing with the most extreme hazard first.

Procedure for Personnel Decontamination

1. Remove contaminated clothing.
2. Wet hands and apply a mild soap or detergent.
3. Work up a good lather with plenty of water.
4. Wash the lather onto the contaminated area for 2 or 3 minutes, being careful not to spread it to other areas.
5. Rinse thoroughly with warm water.
6. Monitor the contaminated area with a survey meter.
7. If necessary, repeat the procedures three or four times, taking care not to scratch or abrade the skin.
8. A moisturizing cream may be applied to prevent chapping.

Procedure for Minor-Spill Decontamination

1. Wash the hands first if they are contaminated as a result of the spill. Finish the cleanup with gloves on the hands.
2. Cover liquid spills with absorbent material to limit the spread of contamination.
3. Other personnel should shut off fans, ventilators, and air conditioners.
4. Mark the contaminted area and restrict the flow of traffic until the cleanup is complete.
5. Be certain that personnel who are leaving the area are not contaminated.
6. If a spill is significant, although this is unlikely with RIA procedures, notify the radiation safety officer.
7. Start decontamination procedures as soon as possible. Normal laboratory cleaning agents will suffice, although specific radiation cleanup agents are available. Begin at the periphery of the area and work inward.

5
Hematology

In the hematology laboratory, you may not see compressed gases, biosafety cabinets, fume hoods, extensive use of flammables, or the blinking and beeping of large pieces of electronic instruments. You will see hematologists engaging in microscope work, staining slides, performing coagulation studies, and operating Coulter counters on a seemingly endless supply of whole-blood specimens. True, the ever-present hepatitis hazard exists here, but through common sense, an awareness of accident potential, and some general but strictly enforced safety rules, hematology is not a hazardous laboratory occupation.

Each safety-conscious hematology laboratory should have several well-labeled impervious containers for the discard of needles, blades, and glassware. Xylene and other volatiles should be kept where there is good ventilation or directly under the fume hoods (Figs. 5-1 and 5-2). A clean, well-ordered workspace should be required of every technician. Specimens received in hematology are whole blood and not serum, so icteric serum cannot provide a hepatitis warning to the hematologists. Samples from suspected hepatitis patients should, therefore, be well labeled; *all* blood specimens must, of course, be treated with caution. Accidents in hematology most often involve needle sticks, glassware

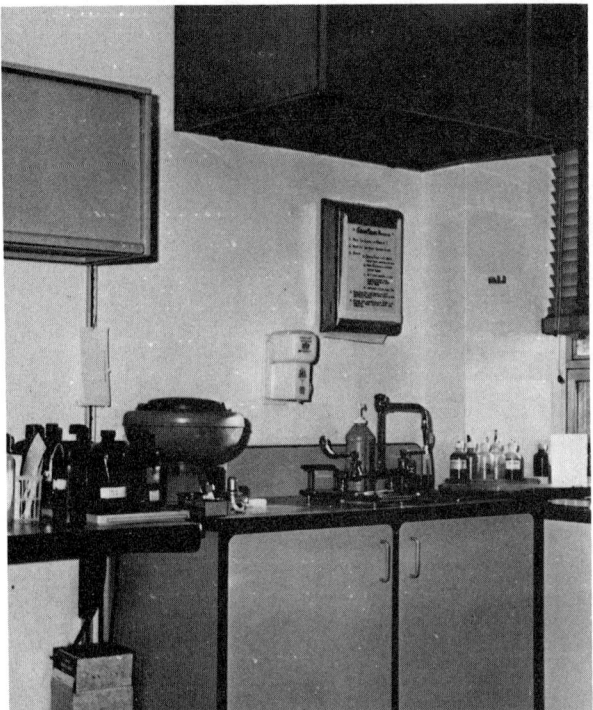

Fig. 5-1. Small amounts of staining materials may be stored and used under the hood.

cuts, and problems arising during venipunctures, so care should be exercised to avoid these incidents.

The hazards and accidents described are all easily avoided by the careful and well-trained hematologist. However, there are hazards that occasionally occur in hematology and other laboratories that are a surprise to those involved and require some entirely new procedure or corrective engineering. This chapter includes such a problem as an illustration of the seriousness of these unexpected but dramatic accidents. Often, drastic measures are necessary to publicize and correct these problems when they occur. This chapter begins with a list of the rules to be followed in the hematology laboratory and then presents a discussion of the hazards and decontamination procedures for sodium azide waste disposal. The chapter concludes with a section on accidental "needle sticks" and an extensive discussion of hepatitis—the virus, the disease and the recommended preventive measures, including valuable information on *Heptavax*-B, the new hepatitis B vaccine. A brief introduction to acquired immune deficiency syndrome (AIDS) is also provided because indications are that it may be a bloodborne disease.

Good Laboratory Practices for the Hematology Laboratory

- Take extreme care when handling and disposing of needles, blades, and glassware. Discard containers must be impervious and must be autoclaved or incinerated before disposal.
- Wear laboratory coats at all times.
- All mouth pipetting is forbidden. Powders for stains and for

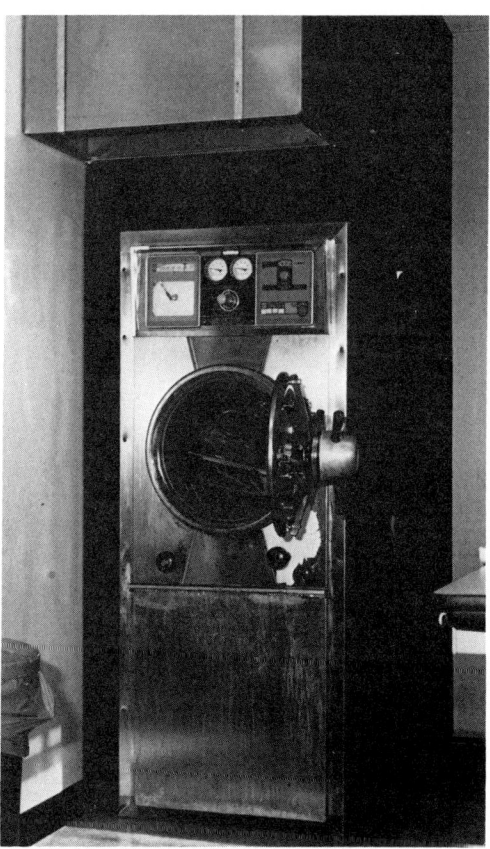

Fig. 5-2. Hazardous products may be released during autoclaving. This autoclave is properly located under a ventilation hood.

coagulation and blood studies must, therefore, be reconstituted with a bulb on the pipette.

- To protect the hands, wear gloves when doing stain preparations.
- If xylene is used for slide clearing, store it under the fume hood or in a well-ventilated area.
- Use only diluent that is free of sodium azide in the Coulter counters.
- For alcohol-based stains, keep the alcohol in metal safety cans.
- If acetone is used for cleaning pipettes, keep it away from flames and store it under the sink.
- Use a small pilot-light flame for sealing the ends of the micro-hematocrit tubes. Use this flame only as required each day, and do not leave it unattended or use it near flammables.
- Wash hands often and *especially* between venipunctures.
- Allow puncture wounds to bleed freely and then rinse them with alcohol to encourage bleeding and help disinfect the area.
- Report *all* accidents (*e.g.,* puncture wounds, glassware accidents) to the supervisor or the employee health unit.
- Use only needle-locking syringes or one-piece needle–syringe units.
- Use a multidraw needle sleeve; it will prevent leaking of blood when several tubes of blood are drawn and will thereby minimize contact between the technologist and the patient's blood.
- Proper waste disposal is important—autoclave or incinerate everything that has contained blood or come into contact with blood (*e.g.,* collection tubes, analysis tubes).
- To avoid aerosol creation, carefully remove the blood-tube caps from the vacuum tubes, pointing them away from the technicians' faces.
- For personnel spills, wash the affected skin with soap and water. Wash any spills on surfaces with an approved, strong disinfectant solution.
- After spinal-fluid counts, decontaminate the chamber overnight, then rinse it with methanol and water before reusing. Without this disinfecting, the cerebrospinal fluid (CSF) chamber may contaminate the fingers with dangerous CSF-borne infectious agents.
- Handle suspected carcinogens, such as formaldehyde, as cautiously as you would known carcinogens. This requires extra

awareness when using a suspected carcinogen: cover suspect containers when not in use. Do not inhale the suspected carcinogen. Special waste disposal is often required. Rinse well if the suspected carcinogen comes into contact with the skin or the work surface.

- Use a commercial cleaner, rather than xylene, to clean microscope slides. Keep xylene in a glass container with a lid and keep the lid on when not using the xylene.
- If a hot plate is used for special stains, warn others that it is on and stay with the hot plate when it is in use. Allow it to cool in a safe place and flag it so that others will not be burned.
- Use microscopes with well-adjusted optics to avoid eye strain.

THE AZIDE HAZARD—A LESSON ON WASTE DISPOSAL

History

Sodium azide was formerly used in large quantities in a number of laboratory procedures, most significantly as the diluent Isoton in automated blood-cell counters. It is now restricted to use as a preservative in laboratory reagents. By 1976, several violent explosions during routine maintenance of clogged laboratory sinks had caused a nationwide alert to this previously unrecognized waste-disposal hazard. The result was that laboratory sinks and drains were carefully decontaminated, copper or lead traps were replaced by polyvinyl chloride (PVC) or glass traps (Fig. 5-3), and Isoton and other solutions were replaced with azide-free substitutes. The azide-free label should appear on all the fluids used in automated cell counters (Fig. 5-4).

The azide-decontamination methods of the Centers for Disease Control (CDC) are presented here in full, because sodium azide may still persist in some plumbing and be used in some procedures, and because this is a good illustration of a serious and unexpected problem. Although the engineering or maintenance staff *were* and *are* those at highest risk and would likely perform the required decontamination procedures, a lesson will be learned by the medical technologist about complacency and waste disposal.

The azide explosions referred to, occurred in waste-piping systems containing copper, lead, brass, or alloys. These metals reacted with the

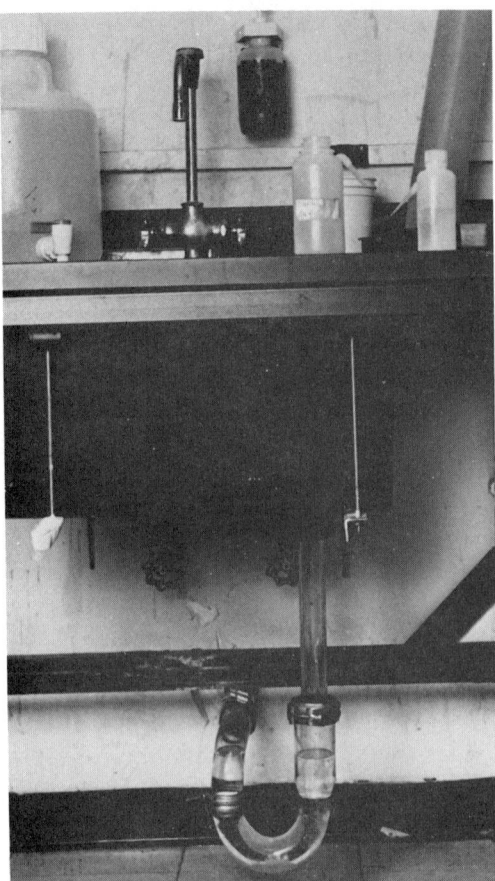

Fig. 5-3. Glass U-tubing has replaced copper U-tubing because a sodium-azide hazard existed.

sodium azide to produce heavy-metal azides. This possibility exists whenever azides are allowed to come into contact with heavy metals. Metal azides are unusually sensitive to mechanical shock; they therefore have exploded violently during routine maintenance such as unblocking of clogged drains. Even nitroglycerin is a less sensitive explosive than are these heavy-metal azide salts (which are used in the explosives industry as detonating agents).

The possibility of an explosive azide may also occur under other laboratory circumstances. An incident was reported in which a violent azide explosion occurred while a constant-temperature water bath, using sodium azide as a preservative, was being repaired. Another potential hazard exists when open containers of sodium-azide solution are stored in refrigerators or cabinets containing exposed copper parts.

It is strongly recommended that those facilities using azide solutions in *any* manner investigate their handling and waste-disposal procedures to eliminate any potentially dangerous conditions.

Neutralization of Sodium-Azide Wastes*

1. If the waste is solid, it is dissolved in enough water to ensure an azide concentration of less than 5%.
2. To this solution, a 20% solution of sodium nitrite ($NaNO_2$) is added until the quantity of sodium nitrite added is 1.5 lb for each pound of sodium azide present. Mix well.
3. Very slowly, and with continuous stirring, a 20% solution of

*As recommended by the Office of Biosafety, Centers for Disease Control, Atlanta, GA.

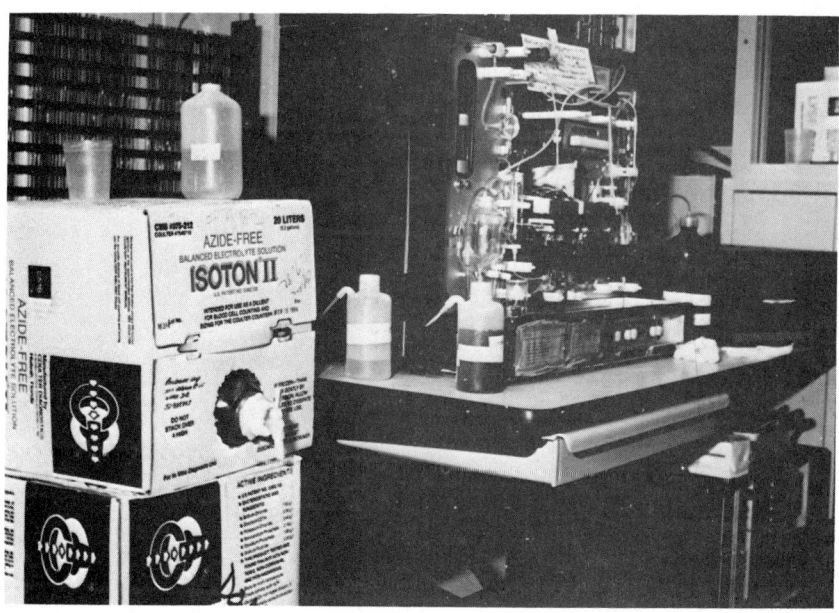

Fig. 5-4. As a result of sodium-azide explosions, automated cell counters now use only azide-free fluids.

sulfuric acid is added until the waste solution is just acid as indicated by litmus. (Caution! Good ventilation is required. Toxic oxides of nitrogen are given off.)
4. When the acidified solution turns starch iodide paper blue, there is excess nitrite present and the decomposition is complete. The waste solution can then be safely discarded through the sewer system.

If the diluting fluid contains 0.1% sodium azide as a preservative, this would amount to about 20 g/5 gal and would require about 30 g of sodium nitrite for decomposition.

Decontamination Procedures for Copper or Lead Plumbing Containing Azides*

1. Prepare 1 liter to 2 liters of 10% w/v sodium hydroxide (100g NaOH/liter of water).
2. Syphon all liquid from the trap and drain using a soft rubber or plastic hose. Use proper precautions against any hazardous chemicals that may be present.
3. Pour the sodium hydroxide slowly into the trap.
4. Tape a Chemical Hazard warning sign to the sink. Write "Do Not Use Sink" on the sign.
5. Allow the solution to remain in the trap a minimum of 16 hours.
6. Flush the drain with water for a minimum of 15 minutes. If the drain will not flow, the sodium hydroxide should be removed by syphoning, if possible, and then diluted with water.

Maintenance Precautions

Because the possibility of residual sodium hydroxide is always present, personnel should wear rubber gloves and face shields when breaking the drain line or trap for maintenance. This equipment should be worn when breaking *any* laboratory drain, because the presence of hazardous chemicals should always be suspected.

*As recommended by the Office of Biosafety, Centers for Disease Control, Atlanta, GA.

General Precautions to Be Followed Where Azides May Be in Use

1. Formation of metallic azides can be minimized by preventing collection of sodium-azide solutions in traps and drains. This can be done by thoroughly flushing drains with water when discarding any solutions containing sodium azide.
2. Deposit azide wastes into a drain that receives plenty of waste water through daily use and periodic flushing. Copious flushing dilutes the azide solution and reduces contact between azides and metal pipes to a minimum. The rapid flow should continue throughout the system, with the final point of discharge being a sewer with a high rate of flow.
3. Install a plastic or glass drain trap and plastic or glass piping next to the trap in any drain into which azide wastes are deposited.
4. Install suitable piping materials in new installations to eliminate potentially dangerous conditions.

ACCIDENTAL NEEDLE STICKS

The most significant occupational disease hazard for medical technologists is hepatitis and, as might be expected, the most prevalent occupational accidents are puncture wounds or needle sticks. The problem of being stuck by used needles is not a trivial one and this occupational hazard is shared by nurses and housekeeping workers.

A May 1981 article stated that in 1980, the University of Virginia Hospital spent $50,000 on 375 people who were accidentally stuck with used needles.* These needle sticks constituted 37% of the total accidents in the hospital that year. Accidental sticking carries with it the threat of hepatitis and, as a result, the hospital spent $40 to $600 on tests and treatments for each employee reporting a puncture accident. Each such incident involves an investigation of the source of the needle as well as blood tests of the victim. Often, when the patient in whom the needle was originally used cannot be identified, the puncture victim is treated with gamma globulin and checked after 3 months and again after 6 months for the development of hepatitis antibodies or antigen in the

*Needlesticks take high toll. The Draw Sheet, p. 30. University of Virginia, 1981.

serum. When the needle has been used in a known hepatitis carrier, two doses of hepatitis B immune globulin are routinely given at a cost of $135 to $165 per dose. The victim in these cases is checked after 3, 6, and 12 months. Now, thanks to a new hepatitis B vaccine approved by the Food and Drug Administration in November 1981, preventive immunization will provide better protection against needle-stick hazards.

Although more nurses and housekeeping staff members suffer these puncture wounds than do medical technologists, these wounds are a most serious hazard for those technicians who draw blood for laboratory tests or use needles in any laboratory procedure. Proper and careful disposal of needles by clipping or discarding into impervious containers easily prevents the majority of these accidents. In addition, no needles or syringes discarded into an impervious container should be finally disposed of until the container has been autoclaved or incinerated. Recapping of used needles is not recommended.

VIRAL HEPATITIS—A LABORATORY HAZARD

Viral hepatitis is the major job-related disease hazard in all clinical laboratories. No laboratory (or technician) that handles blood, blood products, or body fluids of any sort is immune to this risk. Laboratories where blood is collected, needles are used, or puncture hazards exist are at some additional risk and require special precautions. Because hematology technicians often perform venipunctures, the hepatitis discussion is placed in this chapter. All clinical laboratory departments, however, share this occupational risk.

The Virus and Disease (A, B, and Non-A, Non-B)

For the medical technician, the hepatitis viruses of concern appear to be, primarily, hepatitis B virus (HBV) and, secondarily, non-A, non-B hepatitis virus. The severity of the risk to the laboratory worker and the seriousness of the disease require an extensive look at the topic of viral hepatitis. The knowledge thus obtained should serve to heighten the care taken with all blood and blood products as well as everything with which the blood has come into contact.

Hepatitis virus can infect man through two quite different routes:

by ingestion, the fecal–oral route; and by injection, the parenteral route. Formerly, it was thought that there were only two types of hepatitis virus—hepatitis A virus (HAV), or infectious hepatitis, and HBV, or serum hepatitis. It was common knowledge that hepatitis A was contracted by the fecal-oral route and hepatitis B by the parenteral route. Now the picture has become much more complicated and research has raised questions that have yet to be answered. Serotypes of hepatitis B have been discovered, and a very prevalent infectious hepatitis seems to occur that is identified thus far as only non-A, non-B hepatitis. The routes of transmission are now blurred because both HAV and HBV can be obtained in infectious blood through oral *and* parenteral routes. Because of this, it is mandatory that there be no smoking, eating, drinking, or storage of food in laboratories where blood specimens are handled and tests are performed.

All of the hepatitis viruses have been extremely difficult to cultivate in the laboratory or in animal hosts and, therefore, understanding the organism, devising treatments, and establishing prevention strategies often rest on indirect and epidemiologic evidence. It is estimated that acute viral hepatitis of all three types exists at about one to two cases per 1000 in the general population. A significant percentage of patients with acute or chronic hepatitis remains undiagnosed. The disease is communicable in the preclinical and early clinical phases and infectivity may be waning at the time enzyme-detection test results first rise.

Comparison of the Three Hepatitis Viruses

The three viruses, A, B, and non-A, non-B, have nearly the same symptoms and are difficult to distinguish without laboratory tests. Milder cases of the disease and those lacking signs of jaundice are often misdiagnosed as influenza, gastroenteritis, or even infectious mononucleosis. The beginning of the disease state includes malaise, anorexia, nausea, vomiting, fatigue, diarrhea, liver tenderness, and mental depression. Anicteric hepatitis—no jaundice with normally colored serum —is two to three times more common than the icteric forms and thus presents an increasing risk to the laboratory worker who tends to treat only an obviously icteric sample as a hazard. When jaundice becomes evident, the urine also darkens and the feces turn pale. Hepatitis is often milder in children, and many cases in children are anicteric. Mortality ranges from 0.1% to 1% in adults.

HBV is by far the most severe and prolonged of the three viruses, and it is the one that most frequently leads to complications and relapses. HBV is a viral infection of the liver. It can lead to serious and life-threatening acute and chronic liver disease and has been associated with a number of immune-complex diseases.

Epidemiologic surveys by the CDC indicate that about 200,000 HBV infections occur in the United States each year. Of these, about 50,000 patients experience acute hepatitis with jaundice, 10,000 require hospitalization, and 12,000 to 20,000 become HBV carriers (approximately 750,000 total in the United States). Chronic active hepatitis develops in over 25% of carriers. Each year about 4000 deaths due to cirrhosis and 800 deaths due to liver cancer are estimated to be related to chronic HBV infections.

Disease treatment involves primarily rest and restricted diet. Liver-function tests are checked often to prevent the damage that would result from a patient's resuming normal activity too quickly. Most often, no permanent liver damage occurs and, after the fatigue ends, the patient usually recovers completely.

To provide an overview and comparison of the three hepatitis viruses and to let the laboratory worker assess the risks of each virus in his work, Table 5-1 has been compiled.

Hepatitis Antigens, Hepatitis Antibodies, and Heptavax-B

Although research into the three types of hepatitis virus continues, the most information has been gathered about HBV—the most serious disease producer of the three. A wide variety of antigen–antibody systems has been uncovered, electron-microscope visualizations have been performed, and a battery of HBV tests have been developed, although many of these are still research tools and not diagnostically available or useful.

The HBV, also called the Dane particle, has three antigen–antibody systems and one specific enzyme, as described in Table 5-2. With the explanation of hepatitis antigens and antibodies, it is easier to understand the significance and mode of action of the Hepatitis B vaccine, Heptavax-B.

In November 1981, this pure inactivated hepatitis B surface antigen (HB$_s$Ag) vaccine was licensed for use by Merck Sharp and Dohme.

The vaccine is produced from blood containing HB_sAg and provokes an antibody to HB_sAg (anti-HB_s) in recipients (Figs. 5-5, 5-6, 5-7). This confers the same immunity as would a bout with the disease.

Heptavax-B was shown to have a protective efficacy of 92.3% among high-risk populations, preventing both active and asymptomatic infection and the carrier state when three doses of vaccine were administered over a 6-month period. Heptavax-B is the most technically complex of any vaccine and represents a breakthrough in preventive medicine. Safety is assured by the use of three inactivation steps in the vaccine-production process, each of which alone would inactivate any known virus.

Experience with more than 6000 vaccine doses given has revealed no evidence of HBV infection and no significant adverse side-effects Clinical reactions observed have been minimal and transient (*e.g.*, mild local tenderness at the injection site and slight elevation in temperature in about 3% of adults). This vaccine has been called "unique in concept, with a record of remarkable safety and dramatic efficacy."*

Health-care personnel for whom the vaccine is currently recommended are categorized below according to the American Hospital Association's criteria of degree of risk:† Categories 1A and 1B are classified as high risk. Categories 2 and 3, not provided, are moderate- and low-risk categories.

> Category 1A—Persons who have frequent, direct, intense contact with blood or infected tissues, who are at risk of trauma, needle sticks, cuts, and abrasions that may result in HBV infection
> - Surgeons, all
> - Nonsurgical personnel who carry out invasive diagnostic and therapeutic procedures, including endoscopists (gastrointestinal internists), invasive cardiologists, angiographers, and other radiologists performing invasive procedures
> - Anesthesiology staff and ancillary personnel
> - Pathology personnel
> - Blood-bank personnel

(Text continues on p. 146)

*Krugman S: The newly licensed hepatitis B vaccine: Characteristics and indications for use. JAMA 247, No. 14:2012–2015, 1982
†From Hepatitis B vaccination program, a general information paper. Bethesda, U.S. Naval Hospital.

Table 5-1. Comparison of Viral Hepatitis A, B, and, Non-A, Non-B

CHARACTERISTICS	HEPATITIS A	HEPATITIS B	NON-A, NON-B HEPATITIS
Antigen identified	Yes	Yes, First was known as Australia antigen, now called HB_sAg. HB_sAg is basis for hepatitis-associated antigen (HAA) test. Other antigens now known are HB_cAg and HB_eAg	No
Epidemics seen	Yes	No	Probably not
Diagnostic laboratory tests available	Research stage only	Yes (*e.g.*, HAA)	None yet, although blood may be screened for alanine aminotransferase (ALT), also known as serum glutamic-pyruvic transaminase (SGPT)
Fatalities	Almost no chance	Some chance	High disposition to progress to chronic liver disease
Cross-immunity	None conferred	None conferred	None conferred
Onset and incubation	Acute, 2 wk–6 wk	Gradual, 6 wk–6 mo	2 wk–15 wk

USA incidence—% of hepatitis cases annually	25%	50%	Estimated 12%–25% of nonepidemic hepatitis and 90% of posttransfusion hepatitis cases among recipients of volunteer-donor and HB$_s$Ag-negative blood
Chronic carrier state (evidence of infectivity)	None; probably high incidence of anti-HAV antibodies in general population.	5%–10% become carriers. Some HB$_s$Ag positives do not spread disease.	Carrier state is indicated.
Prevention—treatment for contacts	Immune globulin often given to household contacts and others exposed. Diminishes severity of disease, no help after disease onset, anti-HAV prevalent in adults.	November 1981 FDA approved Heptavax-B, expected to be 90% effective. Hepatitis B immune globulin seems to help after exposure and has increased level of anti-HB$_s$Ag.	Sometimes immune globulin may be given before multiple transfusions are administered. Seems to reduce icteric cases and development of non-A, non-B hepatitis.
Increased risk to laboratory workers	Apparently none	Yes, via needle sticks and mucosal surfaces	Yes, via needle sticks and mucosal surfaces
Spread, risks	Spread by direct contact, carried in feces, contaminated food, H$_2$O, and so on. Rarely if ever associated with posttransfusion disease.	Blood, blood products, carriers, close personal contact, sex, saliva, semen, ear piercing, injections, tattoos; drug addicts, blood-bank workers, dialysis center workers, dentists. As little as 0.0000001 ml can infect.	Posttransfusion and unknown
Recommended precautions	Good hygiene, handwashing, personal sanitation	Care with all blood and blood products	Care with all blood and blood products

- Phlebotomists; personnel involved in intravenous therapy
  Category 1B—Persons who have slightly less exposure to
  infected blood than those in Category 1A, but who are never-
  theless in close or direct contact with blood or infected tissues
- Clinical-laboratory technical staff

Table 5-2. Antigens and Antibodies of Hepatitis B Virus

NAME	ANTIBODY–ANTIGEN ABBREVIATION	SIGNIFICANCE
Hepatitis B surface antigen	HB_sAg	Noninfectious, outer viral envelope by itself
Antibody to Hepatitis B surface antigen	Anti HB_s	Exposure to HB_sAg; denotes immunity to reinfection; the protective antibody after Heptavax-B administration When hepatitis B immune globulin is administered, anti-HB_s provides passive protection
Hepatitis B core antigen	HB_cAg	Presence of the disease; not normally tested for
Antibody to Hepatitis B core antigen	Anti-HB_c	Present shortly after HB_sAg, persists for years; alone, does not confer immunity
Hepatitis B e antigen	HB_eAg	Presence denotes continuing inflammatory process
Antibody to Hepatitis B e antigen	Anti-HB_e	Presence indicates marked reduction in degree of infectivity
DNA polymerase	DNA-P	May ultimately be the most sensitive measure of HBV infection

- Respiratory-therapy technicians
- Clinical immunologists
- Nurses in emergency wards, intensive care units, coronary care units, oncology units, operating rooms, obstetric suites, dialysis units, and burn units

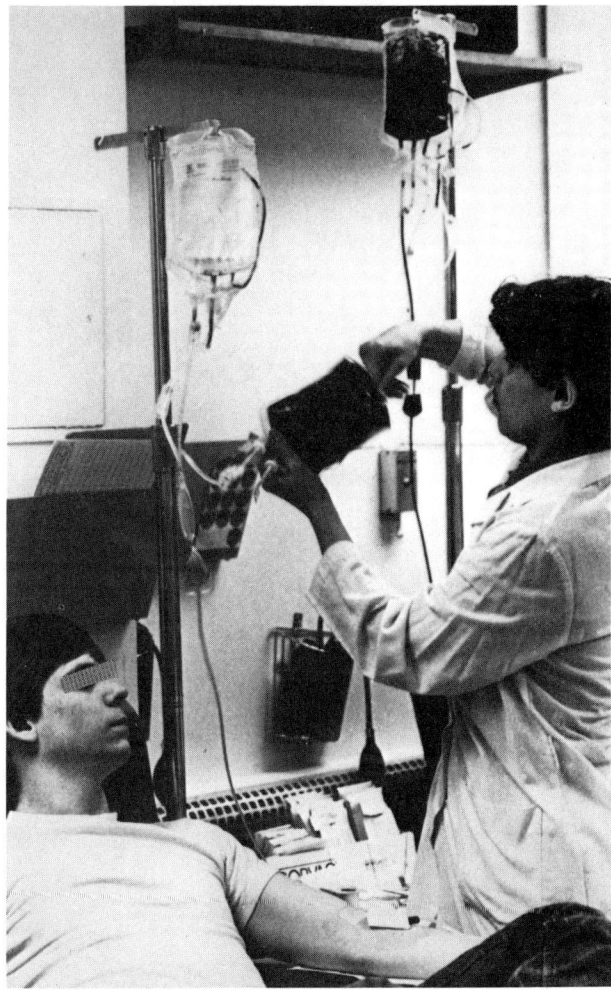

Fig. 5-5. Human plasma containing hepatitis B surface antigen is used to produce Heptavax-B, a vaccine to help prevent hepatitis B infection. A donor is shown here at the New York Blood Center, one of several specially licensed collection centers across the country. (Photo courtesy of Merck Sharp & Dohme)

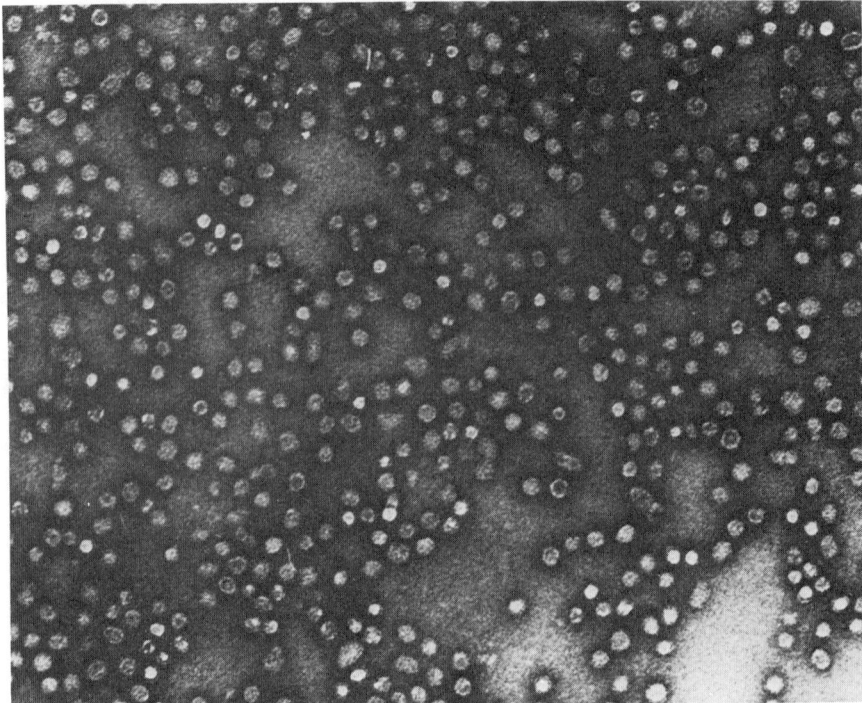

Fig. 5-6. Hepatitis B surface antigen, which is used to manufacture Heptavax-B. (Original magnification × 56,000) (Photo courtesy of Merck Sharp & Dohme)

General Precautions for Prevention of Laboratory-Acquired Viral Hepatitis

These general precautions, when strictly followed, drastically lessen the chances that a medical technologist in a clinical laboratory will acquire hepatitis through his own work habits.

Personal Hygiene

- Wear a laboratory coat at all times.
- Use disposable aprons and gloves as appropriate for procedures.
- Remember that mouth pipetting is not acceptable for any reason.
- Wash hands frequently and thoroughly whether visibly contaminated or not.

- Remember that eating, smoking, and drinking in the laboratory are forbidden.
- Store food only in specially marked refrigerators.
- Keep fingers, pencils, and so on out of the mouth.
- Label hepatitis-positive specimens and keep them in plastic transport bags (Fig. 5-8).

Collection and Processing

- Process blood, especially positive or icteric specimens, over absorbent paper.
- Collect blood from hepatitis-positive patients last, and wear gloves when processing their specimens.
- Avoid the creation of aerosols in all procedures.
- Cap specimens during centrifugation.
- Process hepatitis-positive sera last.

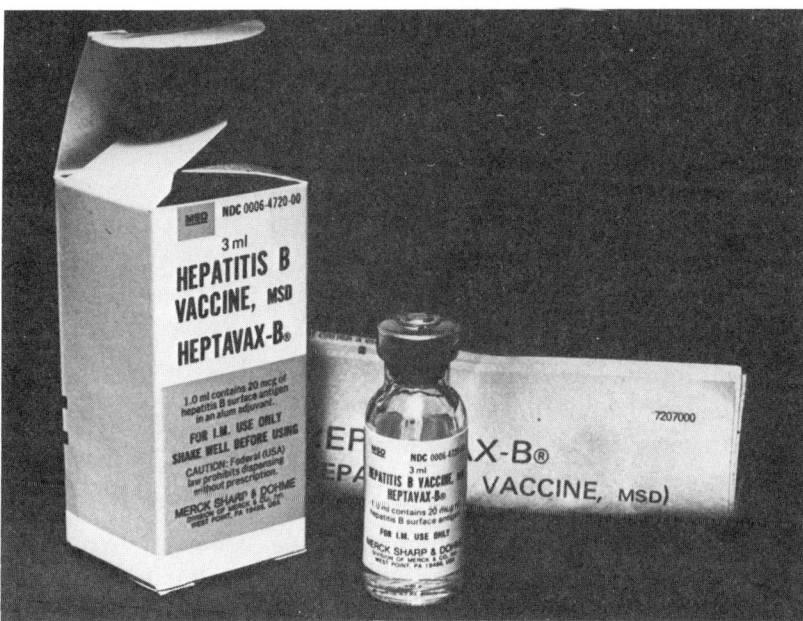

Fig. 5-7. Newly licensed Heptavax-B vaccine promises to provide protection for hepatitis-risk occupations, including those in the clinical laboratory. (Photo courtesy of Merck Sharp & Dohme)

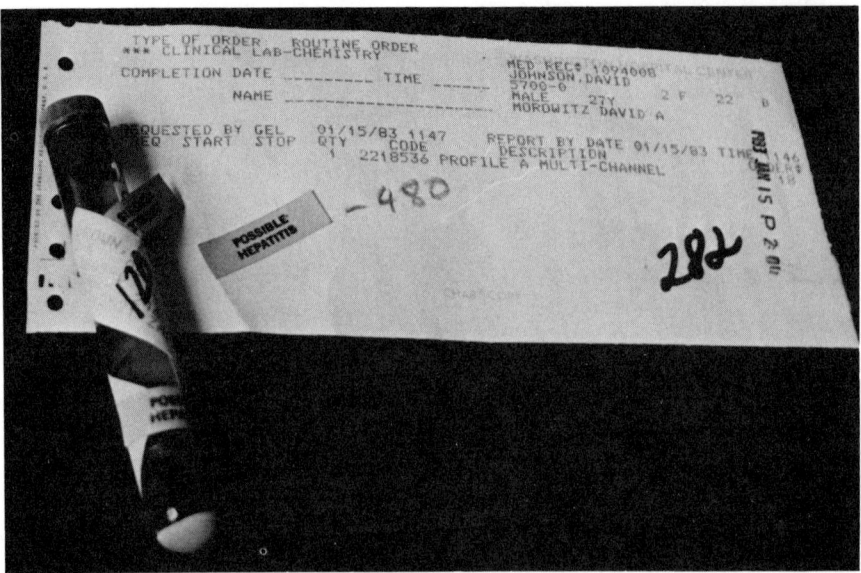

Fig. 5-8. For safety in the laboratory, blood collected from known or suspected hepatitis patients should be specially labeled, as should the requisition slip. Gloves should be worn when this blood is handled and collected.

Work-Area Maintenance

- Keep the work area clean and tidy.
- Avoid the use of pooled human sera in all procedures.
- Use care in the maintenance of instruments.
- Use a strong bleach solution to clean the workbench before and after each shift.
- Flood the work area with bleach solution after spills occur.
- To protect maintenance and housekeeping staffs, dispose of contaminated material properly. This means autoclaving of all biohazardous material.
- Soak laboratory hardware in deep containers filled with bleach.

First Aid After Contamination or Likely Contamination of Personnel

- Wash the skin well with soap and water.
- Notify the physician in charge of the laboratory.
- The administration of hepatitis immune globulin to contaminated

personnel is the decision of the physician director of the occupational medicine service or the laboratory pathologist.

- Fill out an incident report for the health service.
- All laboratory personnel with clinical hepatitis should be reported to the hospital safety officer *and* the local or state health department; duly record all information in the employee health service.
- Laboratory management sets the policy on routine HB_sAg and anti-HB_s testing of personnel for detection of carriers or seroconversions.

Effective Methods of Disinfection and Sterilization for Hepatitis-Associated Specimens and Equipment

Heat

- Boiling H_2O, 100°C; for 10 minutes
- Steam under pressure, 121°C, 15 psi, for 15 minutes
- Dry heat, 160°C, for 2 hours

Chemicals

- Solutions of sodium hypochlorite, 0.5% to 1%, for 30 minutes
- Forty percent aqueous formalin (16% aqueous formaldehyde), for 12 hours
- Twenty percent formalin in 70% alcohol, for 18 hours
- Two percent aqueous alkalinized glutaraldehyde, for 10 hours
- Ethylene oxide gas

AIDS—A NEW HAZARD IN THE LABORATORY?

A relentless "new" disease, acquired immune deficiency syndrome (AIDS), is the object of intense scientific scrutiny by public health officials, and is cause for concern in the clinical laboratory as well. Indeed, it presents concern for the *entire* hospital staff because cases may be hard to diagnose and are beginning to occur in greater numbers.

AIDS is a disease for which the etiology remains elusive, and it as yet has no treatment or cure. It has a 100% mortality rate, with death usually occurring within 2 years of diagnosis. The disease appears to "immunodestroy" the victim, irreversibly attacking helper T cells and possibly B-cell mediators. Patients appear first with a flu-like illness and a generalized lymphadenopathy, often followed soon thereafter with untreatable malignancies, primarily Kaposi's sarcoma. Opportunistic infections with one or several known organism may also appear. In the course of the disease, patients may develop *any* disease and any symptoms, at any time and in any or *every* organ and tissue.

As case numbers begin to grow and a pattern emerges, the population at greatest risk for this disease consists of hemophiliacs, male homosexuals, Haitian entrants to the United States, and intravenous drug abusers. Although other theories of causation exist, opinion seems to favor the theory that the responsible factor is transmissible and infectious, presumably a virus, and can contaminate blood and blood products. Voluntary or compulsory exclusion of high-risk groups from blood donation is one suggested preventive measure. Testing blood donors for a "surrogate agent"—probably the anti-HB_c—as a marker is another. The populations at risk for HBV and AIDS overlap considerably.

Why are clinical laboratory employees at any increased risk of contracting this disease? The answer is twofold: if AIDS is a blood-borne disease, the laboratory handles a high volume of blood and blood products; and also subclinical and diagnosed AIDS patients are appearing in increasing numbers in hospitals for treatment and diagnosis. They represent a direct route of person-to-person contact, especially *before* diagnosis is made.

Because the Heptavax-B is made from blood pooled from male homosexuals, among others, and from chronic HB_sAg carriers, initially there was some concern that the vaccine presented an increased AIDS risk. However, there is no evidence to support this concern and, indeed, large numbers of vaccine doses have been given with no ill effects. To date, no person has ever contracted the disease without a history of needle usage, transfusion, or intimate physical contact with an AIDS patient.

In three Heptavax-B–placebo trials between 1978 and 1981 and in an additional 17,602 Heptavax-B recipients throughout 7 years of clinical trials, *no* AIDS was reported. The 65-week-long vaccine preparation employs a triple inactivation process which kills all transmissible agents known. The population at increased risk of contracting HBV is strongly encouraged to take Heptavax-B.

Although there is no evidence of AIDS transmission to hospital personnel from contact with affected patients or clinical specimens, prudence dictates the adoption of the same procedures used for hepatitis patients and specimens. All laboratory personnel must avoid direct contact of skin and mucous membranes with blood, blood products, excretions, secretions, and tissues of persons likely to have AIDS.

The AIDS precautions for laboratory staffs are presented in full in the list below. Additional precautions may be added by each hospital.

The following precautions are advised for persons performing laboratory tests or studies on clinical specimens or other potentially infectious materials (*e.g.,* inoculated tissue cultures, embryonated eggs, animal tissues) from known or suspected AIDS patients:*

- Mechanical pipetting devices should be used for the manipulation of all liquids in the laboratory. Mouth pipetting should not be allowed.
- Laboratory coats, gowns, or uniforms should be worn while working with potentially infectious materials and should be discarded appropriately before leaving the laboratory.
- Gloves should be worn to avoid skin contact with blood, specimens containing blood, blood-soiled items, body fluids, excretions, and secretions, as well as surfaces, materials, and objects exposed to them.
- All procedures and manipulations of potentially infectious material should be performed carefully to minimize the creation of droplets and aerosols.
- Biological safety cabinets (Class I or II) and other primary containment devices (*e.g.,* centrifuge safety cups) are advised whenever procedures are conducted that have a high potential for creating aerosols or infectious droplets. These include centrifuging, blending, sonicating, vigorous mixing, and harvesting infected tissues from animals or embryonated eggs. Fluorescent activated cell sorters generate droplets that could potentially result in infectious aerosols. Translucent plastic shielding between the droplet-collecting area and the equipment operator should be used to reduce the presently uncertain magnitude of this risk. Primary containment devices are also used in handling

---

*Centers for Disease Control: Acquired immune deficiency syndrome (AIDS) precautions for clinical and laboratory staff. Morbid Mortal Wk Rep 31, No. 43, 1982

materials that might contain concentrated infectious agents or organisms in greater quantities than expected in clinical specimens.

- Extraordinary care must be taken to avoid accidental wounds from sharp instruments contaminated with potentially infectious material and to avoid contact of open skin lesions with materials from AIDS patients (Fig. 5-9).
- Blood and other specimens should be labeled prominently with a special warning, such as "Blood Precautions" or "AIDS Precautions." If the outside of the specimen container is visibly contaminated with blood, it should be cleaned with a disinfectant (such as 1:10 dilution of 5.25% sodium hypochlorite [household bleach] with water). All blood specimens should be placed in a second container, such as an impervious bag, for transport. The

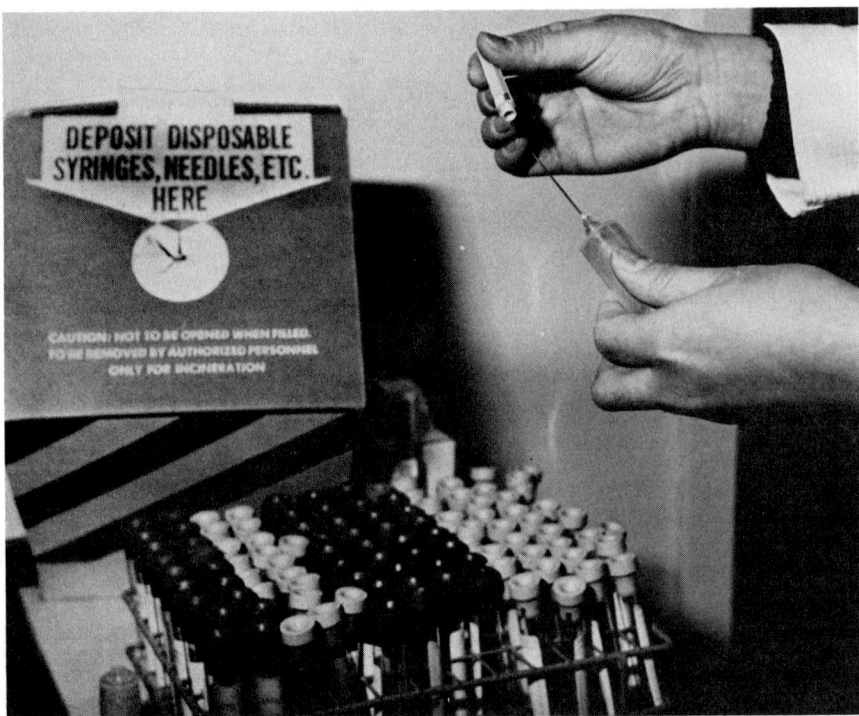

Fig. 5-9. Laboratory policy may vary as to capping or clipping of needles. Capping, as seen here, presents an obvious risk of self-puncture to the technician.

container or bag should be examined carefully for leaks or cracks.

- Articles soiled with blood should be placed in an impervious bag prominently labeled "AIDS Precautions" or "Blood Precautions" before being sent for reprocessing or disposal. Alternatively, such contaminated items may be placed in plastic bags of a particular color designated solely for disposal of infectious wastes by the hospital. Disposable items should be incinerated or disposed of in accord with the hospital's policies for disposal of infectious wastes. Reusable items should be reprocessed in accord with hospital policies for HBV-contaminated items. Lensed instruments should be sterilized after use on AIDS patients.
- Needles should not be bent after use, but should be promptly placed in a puncture-resistant container used solely for such disposal (Fig. 5-9). Needles should not be reinserted into their original sheaths before being discarded into the container, because this is a common cause of needle injury.
- Disposable syringes and needles are preferred. Only needle-locking syringes or one-piece needle–syringe units should be used to aspirate fluids from patients, so that collected fluid can be safely discharged through the needle, if desired. If reusable syringes are employed, they should be decontaminated before reprocessing.
- Laboratory work surfaces should be decontaminated with a disinfectant, such as sodium hypochlorite solution, following any spill of potentially infectious material and at the completion of work activities.
- All potentially contaminated materials used in laboratory tests should be decontaminated, preferably by autoclaving, before disposal or reprocessing.
- All personnel should wash their hands following completion of laboratory activities, following removal of protective clothing, and before leaving the laboratory.

6
Microbiology

In the summer of 1975, before its new quarters opened, a large hospital in the Washington area housed many of its clinical laboratories in makeshift quarters that had been converted from previous non-laboratory use. The microbiology laboratory, located at the back of one low-rise building adjacent to the hospital, provided a setting that should no longer be found in *any* clinical laboratory. A brief description illustrates: Microbiology specimens were dropped off at a collection desk in the front of the building; few specimens, if any, were rejected, and many were leaking or poorly labeled. The technologists went to the desk to pick up their specimens whenever time permitted. This meant that some specimens were cultured rapidly and others were not.

The microbiologists worked at assigned work benches in the main "micro" laboratory, where the incoming plating bench was just a few feet from both the busy open door and the coffee area. The coffee area had only an upholstered bench and a laboratory chair or two as needed. There was also a table with a hot-water pot, instant coffee, tea, and soup ingredients belonging to the staff. Many birthday cakes and cold drinks were dispensed from this table and a variety of knives and forks were kept for such occasions. In fact, no other eating space was available in the entire laboratory building. Eating and drinking were often not strictly limited to the coffee area when several people took a break together and visits spilled over into the work area.

In the routine micro laboratory, mouth pipetting was commonplace and inoculating loops were flamed before and after use on open Bunsen burners, as were the lips of test tubes. A refrigerator stored lunch items and various "clean" laboratory materials. Everyone wore government-issue laboratory clothing if they so chose, and free laundering was available. Bare feet in sandals were the choice of the women for both summer coolness and an easy lunchtime tan. Contaminated plates were thrown into large steel buckets and were carried, usually two buckets at a time, overflowing when full, down the hall to the autoclave room. *No* routine work was performed under a hood. Precautions for tuberculosis and mycology were somewhat more strict and masks were worn for safety during tuberculosis (TB) procedures. Several accidents that summer in the TB-laboratory centrifuge resulted in aerosol contamination of the entire laboratory and the ventilation system. When the aerosol had settled sufficiently for the staff to resume work, the workers were required to wear masks for the remainder of those days. Chest x-rays and tine tests were given to everyone who had been present when the accidents occurred. No one contracted a laboratory-acquired infection all of that summer . . . or did they?

These descriptions are accurate, but memories dim somewhat over the years. Conditions were probably even a bit more shocking than this brief description recalls. What *is* important is the change that has occurred in the laboratory in such a short period of time. Although medical technologists personally should never be subjected to working conditions such as these, they should all be able to recognize the potential hazardous conditions just described and should be fully aware of the preventive measures now used. The vigilance required in a laboratory where one is surrounded by infectious agents remains, but the option to work in a manner that endangers oneself or others is no longer acceptable.

Although infectious disease is obviously present in hospital patients, it may not be so obvious that the causative organisms can be easily spread to the clinical laboratory where workers test blood and body fluids from these infected patients. Often infectious-patient samples are not identified as such, or an infection may exist in a subclinical state in patients admitted for other causes. As a result, the microbiology laboratory handles specimens of initially unknown biological hazard and must, for identification, isolate and grow organisms in millions per milliliter. Additionally, there is no control over the physical form of the organisms (*e.g.,* spores, toxins) encountered. As should be readily apparent, safety precautions are the only solution to working with these hazarads while maintaining the health of the microbiology staff.

The purpose of this chapter is to alter the odds at work against the microbiologist by identifying those sources of biological hazard (biohazard) that are not always readily apparent. The chapter begins with rules of good laboratory practice for the microbiology laboratory; these must be adhered to *without exception*. The benefits should be obvious.

The hazards of aerosol production and laboratory-acquired infections, as well as the mechanisms of employee infection, are discussed in the next section. This is followed by a section on employee protection from the patient in isolation. TB and mycology are treated as special hazards and are presented separately from routine microbiology procedures. Other hazards, spills, contaminated waste, biosafety principles, and containment equipment are covered in some detail. The chapter concludes with the U.S. Department of Health and Human Services' Classification of Etiologic Agents on the Basis of Hazard and a listing of Agents of Disinfection, Sterilization, and Antisepsis; these lists are presented for review and reference.

Good Laboratory Practices for the Microbiology Laboratory

- Handle all blood, body fluids, and stool and urine specimens as if they are contaminated.
- Keep the laboratory doors closed when working to prevent drafts and contamination of other areas.
- Decontaminate work surfaces before work starts, after work is completed, and after spills, using Staphene, Wescodyne, or 70% ethyl alcohol.
- Decontaminate all contaminated waste, including specimens and inoculated material, preferably by autoclaving before further disposal into sinks, waste containers, or the glassware washroom.
- Remember that absolutely *no* mouth pipetting of any kind is permitted.

- Remember that no food, drink, smoking, application of cosmetics or food storage is permitted in the work area.
- Wash hands frequently (especially after handling contaminated material and before leaving the laboratory) with an antiseptic soap containing an antibacterial agent (*e.g.,* iodophor or hexachlorophene).
- Avoid putting fingers, pencils, or other objects into the mouth.
- Continually take care not to create aerosols in any procedure, whether you are opening specimen caps or streaking plates.
- Wear laboratory coats or uniforms in the work area and remove them when leaving for nonlaboratory areas such as the lunchroom.
- You may perform procedures with inactivated antigens on the open bench.
- To minimize the hazard for cleanup or disaster crews, place all biohazardous materials into an appropriately marked refrigerator or incubator at the close of each workday.
- If the autoclave is not located in the laboratory, put contaminated material into a sturdy leakproof bag and seal it for transport to the autoclave.
- Remember that all spills, accidents, and potentially hazardous exposures should be reported to the supervisor and properly recorded and treated.
- Ideally, the laboratory should be designed with impervious, resistant bench tops for ease of cleaning.
- Whenever possible and especially when aerosols are a danger, perform work over plastic-backed absorbent toweling.
- Remember that the microbiology laboratory's handwashing sink should be operated by a foot or elbow control and should not be used as a general waste-disposal site.
- Keep soap and disinfectant (*e.g.,* Hibiclens) readily available at the sink.
- Periodically check, clean, and defrost refrigerators, deep freezers, and ice chests. Keep all refrigerated material well labeled and periodically check it for breakage. Do not store flammable solutions in nonexplosiveproof refrigerators.
- Make sure that water baths contain a disinfectant that is changed and replenished at proper intervals.

- Do not allow visitors or young children to enter the laboratory without special permission.
- Biological safety is the responsibility of the section head.
- Do not put tube cultures upright in cups or beakers; to prevent accidents, always use proper tube racks.
- Do not accept grossly contaminated specimens. If one has been accepted, put the leaking specimen and specimen slip into a clear plastic bag. Recopy the slip, attach it to the outside of the bag, and wash hands well. While wearing gloves, transfer the specimen to the new container.
- Remember that all specimens from patients with isolation precautions should be double-bagged in plastic and labeled *contaminated.*
- Personnel with open cuts should not handle contaminated material without a Band-Aid over the cut, and gloves over that if the procedure involves significant risk.
- Inoculate cultures of highly virulent materials and handle them in a biological safety cabinet.
- Keep the laboratory under negative pressure as compared with the hallway. A small piece of paper tissue held at the half-open door can easily test pressure difference.
- Make sure that specimens known to be infectious are red-tagged when brought to the laboratory.
- Keep inoculation-loop use minimal. Instead, use disposables and applicator sticks whenever possible and drop into a disinfectant (*e.g.,* Wescodyne) after use.
- Use the Bacti-Cinerator to heat all inoculating loops (Fig. 6-1).
- Place pipettes horizontally in a pan of disinfectant. Seal them when full and autoclave them. Do not drop them into an upright cylinder of disinfectant.

Biological Hazard Symbol

All areas and equipment used for biohazardous-material handling or storage should be marked with the biohazard caution sign (Fig. 6-2). Decontaminate the area and remove these signs when the area is no longer used for this purpose. No foodstuffs may be stored in *any* biohazard refrigerator.

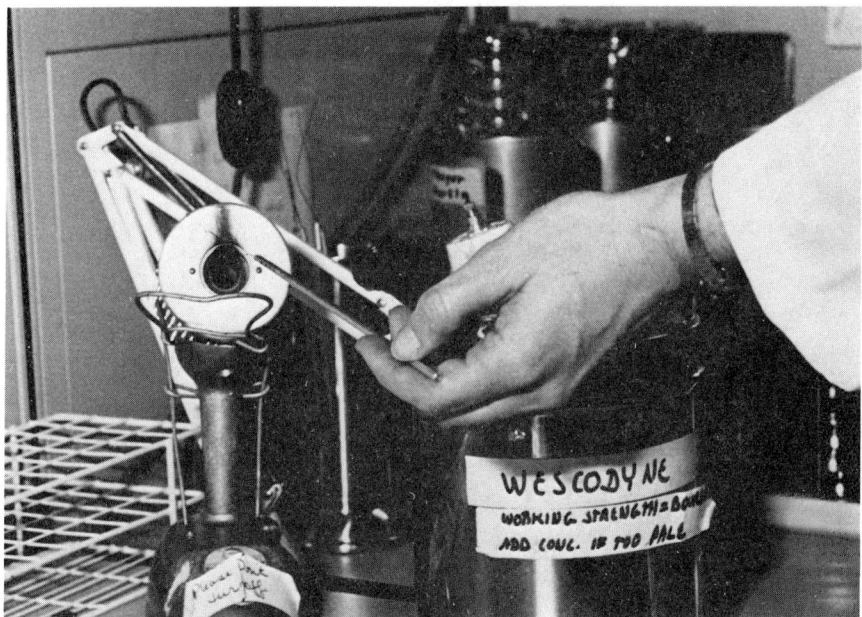

Fig. 6-1. In microbiology, use of a device such as the Bacti-Cinerator for flaming loops eliminates one source of aerosol hazards.

HAZARDS

Aerosol Production and Infection Hazard

Studies have shown that fewer than 20% of laboratory-associated infections may be attributable to known causes such as accidents (Table 6-1). This leaves a surprising number, more than 80%, attributable to unknown causes. However, because there is no universal requirement for reporting laboratory accidents or laboratory-acquired infections, the actual incidence is very likely far greater than published studies indicate. The statistics in these studies were derived from all types of laboratory settings. Research laboratories appear to be the most hazardous; diagnostic- and teaching-laboratory data combined account for about 20% of the total number of laboratory-acquired infections studied. Current scientific thought on the unknown-cause infections

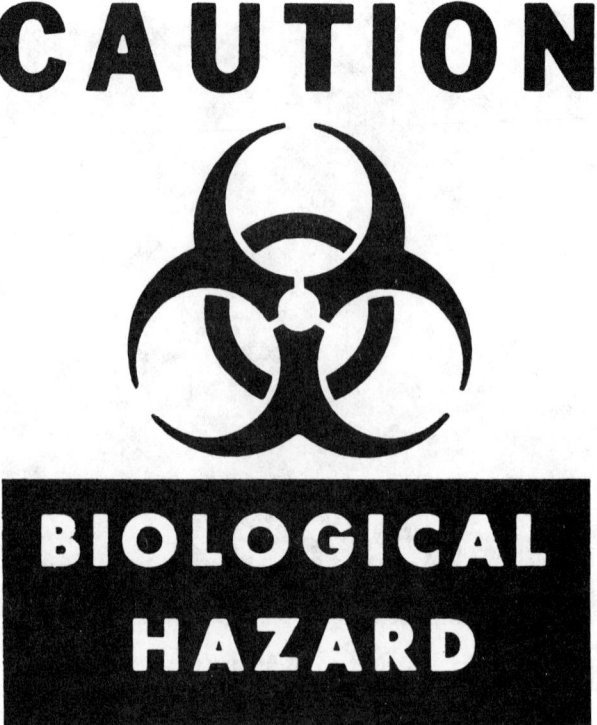

CAUTION

BIOLOGICAL HAZARD

Fig. 6-2. Biological-hazard symbol (biohazard symbol).

attributes the bulk of them to routine microbiological procedures that result in the production of microbe-containing aerosols that go unnoticed by the laboratory worker. The production of these infectious aerosols is a very significant problem in the laboratory. This hazard must be identified and minimized whenever possible because virtually *all* laboratory procedures produce aerosols (Tables 6-2 and 6-3). Indeed, laboratory staffs must increase their abilities to recognize aerosol and accident potentials and to be flexible in their work habits. Accidents do occur more frequently when regulations are knowingly violated, when work is performed at increased speeds, and during the diluting and plating of cultures. Awareness of these problems should result in extra caution on the part of the medical technologist when aerosols are produced, or if possible, in elimination of those procedures that create aerosols.

Centrifuging represents one of the most obvious aerosol-creating

Table 6-1. Most Common Causes of Accidental Laboratory Infections by Percentage

CAUSE	PERCENTAGE OF INFECTIONS*
Oral aspiration through pipette	4.7
Accidental syringe inoculation	4.0
Animal bite	1.4
Spray from syringe	1.2
Centrifuge accident	0.2
Subtotal	12.0
Unknown (possible causes—cuts or scratches from contaminated glassware, spilling or splattering of pathogenic cultures, creation of infectious aerosols)	88
Total	100.0

*From a study of 3700 infections. (Adapted from NIH Biohazards Guide, 1974)

Table 6-2. Common Sources of Infectious Aerosols and Recommended Control Measures

SOURCE OF AEROSOL PRODUCTION	AEROSOL-CONTROL MEASURES
Streaking agar plates	Use only smooth agar
Inoculating culture with hot loop	Use only cool loops
Blowing out last drop in pipette	Drain out last drop in pipette
Mixing a culture with pipette	Use a tube mixer
Drop falling on hard work surface	Work over disinfectant gauze
Withdrawing needle from stoppered vaccine bottle	Use alcohol pledget around needle
Using high-speed blender, vortex, or shaking machines to mix sample	Let sample settle 1 hr before opening
Having broken tube in centrifuge	Use safety cups
Removing bubbles from syringe	Drain into alcohol pledget
Heating contaminated inoculating loop	Always use Bacti-Cinerator
Breaking moisture film on Petri plate	Open carefully away from face

Table 6-3. Sources of Aerosol Production in Laboratory Procedures

TYPE OF AEROSOL	PROCEDURE THAT PRODUCES AEROSOL
Surface contamination (>5 μm) Large, settle fast, contaminate work surface and skin	Opening containers Using pipettes (no visible spill) Using test-tube mixers Opening lyophilized cultures Centrifuging
Droplet nuclei (<5 μm) Remain in air, random drift	Careful pouring Using fixed-volume automatic pipettors Pipette mixing of fluid culture Using high-speed blenders Harvesting (dropping infected eggs) Using paint-shaking machines Having pipette spills Dropping tubes or flasks of cultures

Adapted from CDC Laboratory Update 78–37.

procedures in the laboratory and, therefore, one that can be avoided by use of a few simple precautionary measures. To avoid aerosol creation, centrifuging must always be performed with crack-free tubes, and decanting from centrifuge tubes must be avoided. If this cannot be avoided, wipe the rim with a disinfectant. Never fill centrifuge tubes to within 0.5 cm of the rim. Open specimens or cultures should only be centrifuged after they are capped, parafilm covered, or in safety cups. Once breakage has occurred in a centrifuge, the aerosol should be given time to settle before the centrifuge is opened and the damage assessed. Never shake broth cultures so that the plug or cap gets wet, because the plug or cap can spread droplets both in the centrifuge and out.

Laboratory-Acquired Infections

The organisms that most often cause laboratory-acquired infections of both known and unknown origins are *Brucella*, *Salmonella typhi*, TB, *Francisella tularensis*, *Rickettsia*, Q fever, and hepatitis (see the list below and Table 6-4). The highly virulent organisms that produce disease with as little as one infective unit (*e.g., F. tularensis*) are the greatest risks to the laboratory technician. The inhalation route of infection is the most frequent and dangerous: 4% of infections acquired this way result in death, 26% in permanent disability, and 70% in total recovery.

THE MOST-FREQUENTLY REPORTED LABORATORY INFECTIONS*

Typhoid
Brucellosis
Tuberculosis
Q fever
Hepatitis
Tularemia
Soviet hemorrhagic fever
Venezuelan equine encephalitis

*From U.S. Department of Health, Education and Welfare: NIH Biohazards Safety Guide. 1974

Table 6-4. Summary of Laboratory-Acquired Infections by Type of Organism

TYPE OF ORGANISM	PERCENTAGE OF LABORATORY- ACQUIRED INFECTIONS
Bacterial	50
Fungal	6
Parasitic	2
Rickettsial	11
Viral	31
Total	100%

*From a study of 2722 cases. (Adapted from NIH Biohazards Safety Guide, 1974)

Mechanisms of Employee Infection

The following mechanisms of employee infection are presented as a review of the factors necessary for a laboratory-acquired infection. The odds of staying infectionfree vary with each technologist, organism, and accident, but all organisms should be treated as the potential pathogens that, given the proper circumstances, they are.

Bear in mind that most pathogenic organisms have a usual route of infection that produces the characteristic disease. Atypical routes of infection and atypical disease are also potential problems. Therefore, caution is encouraged in working with all unknowns and pathogens.

Mechanisms

- *General health or susceptibility*—good health often provides the margin of safety that prevents disease in a potential host.
- *Size of dose*—a large dose of a relatively harmless organism can overcome host defenses.
- *Virulence of organism*—a highly virulent pathogen may cause infection with a single microbial unit.
- *Route of entry*
    Airborne—the greatest hazard to the microbiologist and other medical technologists, owing to the ever-present infectious aerosols and minidroplets
    Ingestion—from mouth pipetting, dirty hands, food, or drink
    Direct inoculation—accidents with needles, syringes
    Skin contact—through intact skin or conjunctiva, small scratches, or cuts on hands or arms
    Vectors—flies, ticks, mosquitoes (not a significant problem in clinical laboratories)

Employee Protection From the Patient in Isolation

The spread of infection to and among hospital personnel from infectious patients can be a serious problem. With a susceptible medical technologist, a source of infection (the patient or contaminated objects), and a means of transmission (direct, as during blood collection, indirect, as in a puncture with a contaminated needle), infection can readily result. The isolation techniques practiced in hospitals are aimed at curbing the transmission factor in the spread of infection and keeping the disease isolated to the original patient. Degrees of isolation have been designated to minimize the general expense and inconvenience that would result from strict isolation for all infectious patients. The isolation rules must be observed and adhered to by each medical technician upon entry into a patient's room.

Isolation categories and procedures are related to the type of infectious disease present. A card with the required entry precautions should be found on the patient's door or at the nearest nursing station. Necessary equipment for personnel use inside the room should be found at the door as well. A blood-collection tray should *never* be taken by a medical technician into an isolation room. For that matter, the blood-collection tray should never be placed on *any* patient's bed. Only the equipment necessary for the laboratory procedure may be taken inside the room, and everything except the specimen itself must then remain in the room for proper disinfection or dispoaal (Fig. 6-3).

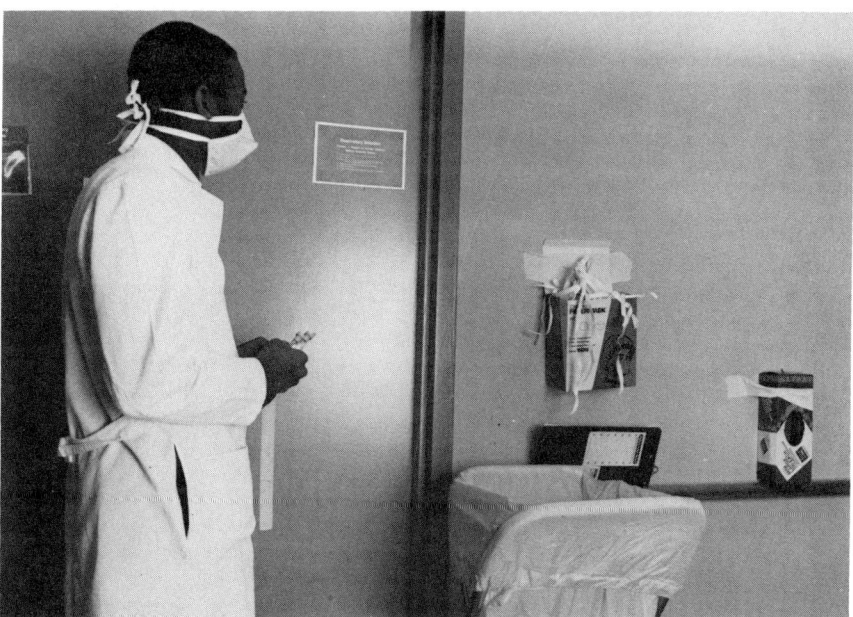

Fig. 6-3. When drawing blood from a patient in isolation, follow all the posted procedures. As a rule, take as little as possible nondisposable equipment into the room.

The following list of commonly designated categories of isolation includes some examples of diseases involved in each type:

- Strict isolation—smallpox, anthrax
- Respiratory isolation—TB, meningitis, measles
- Protective isolation—protects patients with immunosuppression from all potentially opportunistic organisms that may be brought in by others
- Enteric precautions—hepatitis, cholera, *Salmonella*
- Wound and skin precautions—clostridia, group A streptococci, *Staphylococcus aureus*
- Discharge precautions—brucellosis, gonorrhea, Q fever
- Blood precautions—amebiasis, *Clostridium perfringens*, hepatitis

Ideally, the isolated patient is in a private room with a sink, toilet, bath, and good ventilation (six air changes per hour). As required by the type of isolation, mask, gown, cap, and gloves should be put on outside the room, used once, and discarded in the proper container before leaving the room. A sterile gown is only required in protective isolation. The technician's hands should be thoroughly washed with an antiseptic soap, preferably at a sink with a foot or elbow control, after leaving the patient's room. To avoid accidental puncture, the medical technologist should place used and contaminated needles in puncture-resistant containers and should not bend them or try to replace the covers. Laboratory specimens for culture should be placed in transparent double bags so that the contents are visible; they should then be handled as appropriate for contaminated specimens. Especially in hepatitis cases, specimens should be labeled *Contaminated, Hepatitis,* or *Isolation.* Although microbiologists' training allows them to easily accept these procedures, when other, less experienced, personnel short-circuit the requirements, *all* employees are endangered.

The TB and Mycology Laboratories

The TB and mycology laboratories are classified as Class III biohazard areas and require safety precautions even more stringent than those in the general microbiology laboratory (Table 6-5). Sputum

Table 6-5. Summary of Recommended Containment Levels for Infectious Agents

BIOSAFETY LEVEL	PRACTICES AND TECHNIQUES	SAFETY EQUIPMENT	FACILITIES
1	Standard microbiological practices	None—primary containment provided by adherence to standard laboratory practices during open-bench operation	Basic facilities (*e.g.,* school laboratory)
2	Level 1 practices plus wearing of protective gloves and coats when conducting procedures with infectious agents; decontamination of all infectious waste; display of biohazard signs; limited access	Partial containment equipment (*i.e.,* Class I or II biological safety cabinets) used to isolate mechanical and manipulative procedures that produce readily detectable aerosols	Containment facility (*e.g.,* clinical microbiology laboratory)
3	Level 2 practices plus special laboratory clothing; controlled access	Partial containment equipment used to isolate all procedures that may produce aerosols	High-containment facility (*e.g.,* TB and rabies laboratories)
4	Level 3 practices plus entrance through changing room, where street clothing is removed and laboratory clothing donned; shower on exit; all wastes decontaminated on exit from facility	Total containment equipment (*i.e.,* Class III biological safety cabinets) used to isolate all procedures and operations involving infectious materials	Maximum-containment facility (*e.g.,* viral or oncogenic research laboratory)

Adapted from Office of Biosafety: Proposed Biosafety Guidelines for Microbiological and Biomedical Laboratories. Atlanta, Centers for Disease Control.

specimens are often the source of unexpected fungal infections and, for that reason, extreme caution should be exercised during their routine laboratory handling for culture and sensitivity. As a rule, consider these specimens to be contaminated and handle them under a hood or in the TB laboratory.

Suspected *Legionella* is another such hazard. All preparations and examinations of specimens (often lung tissue or aspirates) for *Legionella* species are to be carried out in a biological safety cabinet. The danger of aerosol inhalation while working with the specimen provides a direct mode of entry for the organism into the microbiologist. The following practices must be strictly observed:

Good Laboratory Practices for the TB and Mycology Laboratories

- Perform all TB and mycology work in a biological safety cabinet.
- Limit the work area to laboratory workers only.
- Use TB disinfectant liberally on work surfaces and for immersing the discarded specimens, glassware, and so on (Wescodyne, an iodine derivative, and Amphyl, a phenol derivative, are good disinfectants.)
- Always use capped centrifuge safety cups in the TB laboratory (Fig. 6-4).
- Make sure that the biosafety cabinet is properly and regularly maintained and disinfected according to the manufacturer's instructions.
- Remember that the hospital maintenance crew should not service TB equipment unless they are properly masked, gloved, gowned, and supervised.
- Remove laboratory coats before leaving the TB work area.
- Wear gloves and a mask when working in the TB laboratory.
- Wash hands frequently with a good disinfectant soap such as Hibiclens.
- Heat-fix all TB and mycology smears.
- Culture all sputa from patients, whether identified as normal or suspect, in a TB hood, even if only a routine culture is requested.
- When preparing sputa for TB culture, pour the supernatant into a discard jar that is fitted with a funnel and contains disinfectant.
- Use disposable swabs and discard them after inoculating media.

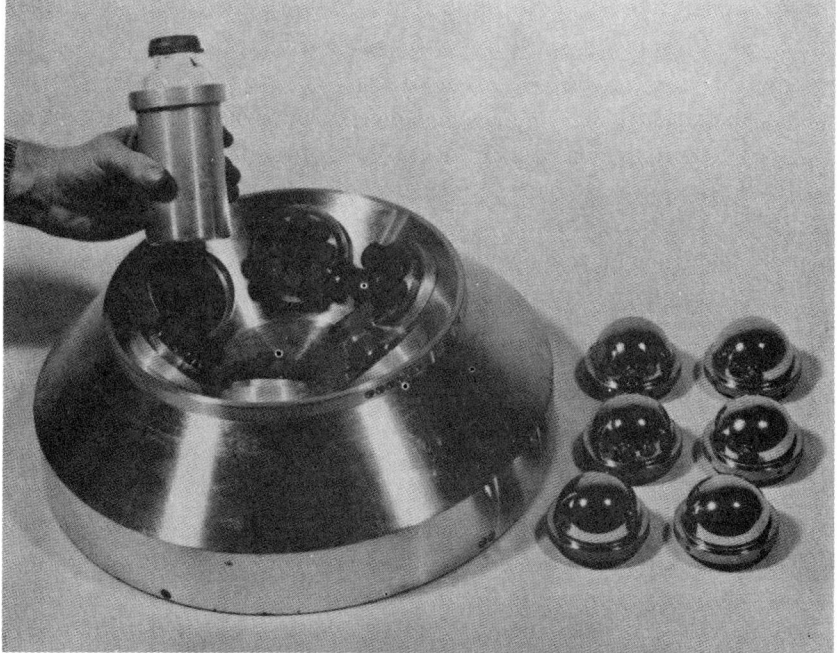

Fig. 6-4. Safety centrifuge cups and caps should always be used when hazard-ous agents are centrifuged or when a hazardous aerosol may be created.

- Clean all work areas carefully when finished.
- Remember that TB workers should be skin tested for TB at the time of employment and annually thereafter.

Other Hazards in the Microbiology Laboratory

Several other hazards may exist in the microbiology laboratory, and these are mentioned briefly:

- Safety procedures for working with *compressed gases* for an-aerobe and CO_2 work can be found in Chapter 7.
- Because *chemical hazards* may also be found in the microbiology laboratory, see the chapter 3 for required precautions.
- *Toxic substances* in disinfectants, such as phenol and iodine, are nonhazardous only at the concentrations found in the working

solutions. The concentrated forms of Wescodyne and Amphyl should *not* be used outside of a fume hood. If only small amounts are needed, only the working solutions should be purchased.

- *Xylene*—only the small amounts required to remove oil from slides should be available in the microbiology laboratory.
- *No open flames* are allowed. The use of alcohol lamps, if permitted by the supervisor, should only take place near the hood. Bunsen-burner use may at times be considered less hazardous than other heat sources (Fig. 6-5).
- *Ether*—only 0.25 lb of ether may be present at one time, for parasite work. It must be stored under or near the hood.
- Because of the volatility or toxicity of *staining ingredients*, stain all slides under the hood.
- Because potential carcinogens are released from the plastic, autoclave *Petri plates* only in autoclaves that are vented to the outside.
- Be alert to the allergic reactions or irritation that may occur in staff members from many *laboratory reagents*—for example, Clorox commonly causes sneezing and contact dermatitis.

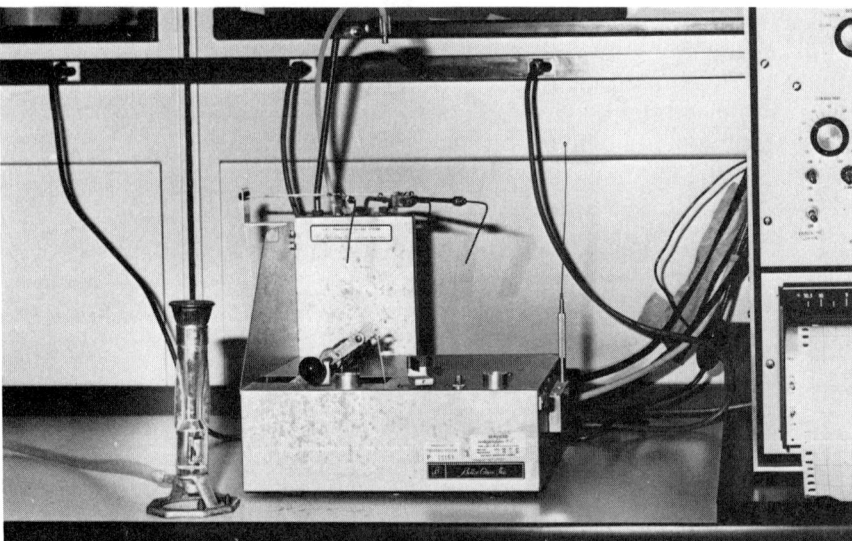

Fig. 6-5. Generally, the use of an open flame is very restricted in the laboratory, although it is still required for some work with anaerobes in microbiology.

Contaminated Waste

The topic of contaminated waste is mentioned throughout other sections of this chapter but is important enough to warrant further attention. *All* wastes containing biohazards should be handled with gloves. Only uncontaminated paper waste such as wrappers, paper towels, and so on may go into the regular waste containers for housekeeping trash removal. All contaminated Petri plates, culture tubes, and so on must be put into autoclavable biohazard bags, sealed with autoclave tape, and autoclaved. The housekeeping staff should not handle the biohazard bags until *after* autoclaving. Swabs and disposables soaked in Wescodyne or a similar disinfectant may be double-bagged and treated with routinely disposed trash. Use stainless-steel trays and pans to soak discards and to transfer contaminated items to the autoclave cart. Again, infectious material must be autoclaved. When using a disinfectant, take care not to splash it. Reusable pipettes should go into dry stainless-steel pans for autoclaving.

TB-laboratory coats, dirty gloves, and even contaminated requisition slips must be autoclaved. To assure adequacy of sterilization, autoclaves require routine testing with spore strips (*Bacillus stearothermophilus*). Never use a shorter cycle time than recommended for autoclaving. Do not leave items to be autoclaved in the autoclave with the intent to autoclave them the next day; someone may accidentally assume they are clean and return them to use, presenting an obvious hazard.

Where biohazardous materials are in use, two separate well-labeled containers or areas should be available. These two areas should be labeled *BIOHAZARDS: TO BE AUTOCLAVED* and *NONINFECTIOUS: TO BE CLEANED.*

Dry hypochlorite or other strong oxidizers should *not* be autoclaved with organics such as paper, oil, and so on. This may be an explosive combination. See Figure 6-6 for a summary of waste handling.

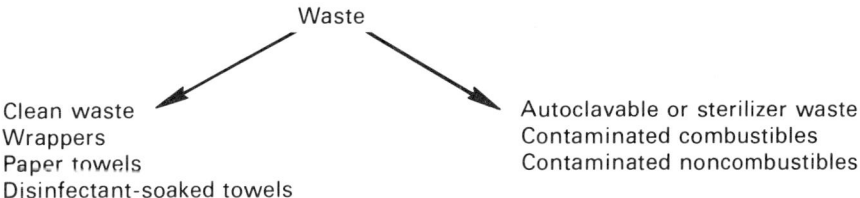

Clean waste
Wrappers
Paper towels
Disinfectant-soaked towels

Autoclavable or sterilizer waste
Contaminated combustibles
Contaminated noncombustibles

Fig. 6-6. All contaminated waste must be autoclaved.

Spills and Accidents (Fig. 6-7)

When an accident involving infectious material occurs, clear the area rapidly and notify the supervisor. Quickly shut down the ventilation system and, if possible, flood the area with a disinfectant. Allow aerosols adequate time to settle and only reenter the contaminated area after half an hour has passed. A gown and mask must be worn during disinfection of the area and cleanup of the spill. Put all cleanup material into biohazard bags for autoclaving. The ventilation system may need to be fogged with a disinfectant to kill aerosolized microbes in the system. Maintenance engineers, *not laboratory staff,* must do this. Baseline serum samples should be obtained from exposed personnel if the situation warrants it.

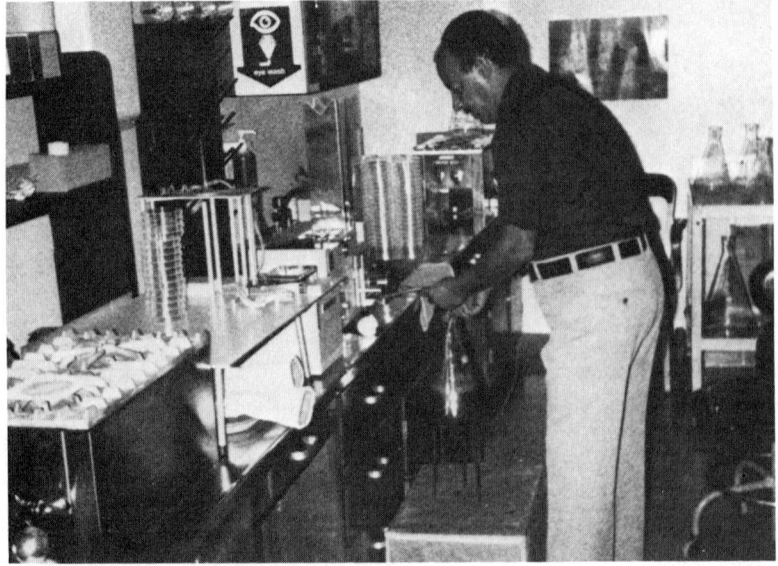

Fig. 6-7. The obvious problems presented with a set-up such as that shown include blockage of the eye wash and materials-spill potential. An inspector would quickly rule this out.

HAZARD PREVENTION

Repairs and Maintenance in the Microbiology Laboratory

All maintenance in the microbiology laboratory should be performed under the supervision of the laboratory supervisor. The maintenance personnel should be given laboratory coats and masks as necessary and should be protected from all laboratory hazards. They are not educated in the same procedures as are the medical technologists and may not be aware of the hazards they will encounter in the laboratory.

Biosafety Principles and Containment Equipment (Table 6-5)

The Centers for Disease Control (CDC) uses the term *containment* in describing methods for managing infectious agents in the laboratory environment where they are being studied, handled or maintained. The following statement is from the CDC's unpublished Proposed Biosafety Guidelines for Microbiological and Biomedical Laboratories:

> . . . primary containment, the protection of personnel and the immediate laboratory environment from exposure to infectious agents, is provided by good microbiological technique and the use of appropriate safety equipment. Secondary containment, the protection of the eternal laboratory environment from exposure to infectious materials, is provided by a combination of facility design and operational practices. The purpose of containment is to reduce exposure of laboratory workers, other persons, and the outside environment to potentially hazardous agents. The three elements of containment include laboratory practices and techniques, safety equipment and facility design.

Generally, the precautions used for the clinical microbiology laboratory should be those required for the agent of highest virulence that may be encountered in the contemplated work. For example, all human sera should be considered potentially infectious for hepatitis, and all sputa should be considered potentially infectious for TB and handled accordingly. When evidence indicates the presence of a single agent of higher or lower risk than expected, procedures can be altered accordingly.

According to the CDC, practices, equipment, and facilities designated as Biosafety Level 2 are

> . . . applicable to clinical, diagnostic, teaching and other facilities working with the broad spectrum of indigenous moderate—risk agents present in the community and associated with human disease of varying severity. Activities with low aerosol potential with these agents can be conducted on the open bench using good microbiological techniques. The hepatitis agents (hepatitis A, hepatitis B, hepatitis non-A, non-B), the salmonellae, and *Toxoplasma* spp are representative of microorganisms assigned to this containment level. Primary hazards to personnel working with these agents relate to accidental auto-inoculation or ingestion of infectious materials. Procedures with high aerosol potential may predictably and significantly increase the risk of exposure of personnel to infectious aerosols and must be conducted in primary containment equipment or devices.

Except for the TB laboratory, which is Class 3, the routine clinical microbiology laboratory is a Class 2 situation.

Biological Safety Cabinets

Biological safety cabinets are microbiological containment equipment specifically designed for the particular type of biohazard that may be encountered in the work (Fig. 6-8). For routine clinical-laboratory hazards, the partial barrier provided by Class I (open-face safety) and Class II (laminar-flow biological safety) cabinets are adequate. Class I cabinets provide only minimal personnel protection; Class II cabinets provide work or personnel protection from low- or moderate-risk biohazards. The Class III (gas-tight biological safety) cabinet provides the highest level of protection attainable for personnel and the environment and is not required in the clinical laboratory.

After installation, a biological safety cabinet must be certified to be working properly and recertified at least every 6 months thereafter. Safety cabinets must be well maintained and checked frequently to determine the adequacy of air flow. They should be washed down frequently; remember that disinfectants do *not* sterilize the cabinet. The ultraviolet (UV) lights used in the biosafety cabinets should be metered for effectiveness at 3-month intervals. UV light should not be turned on when personnel without eye protection are doing manipulations in the

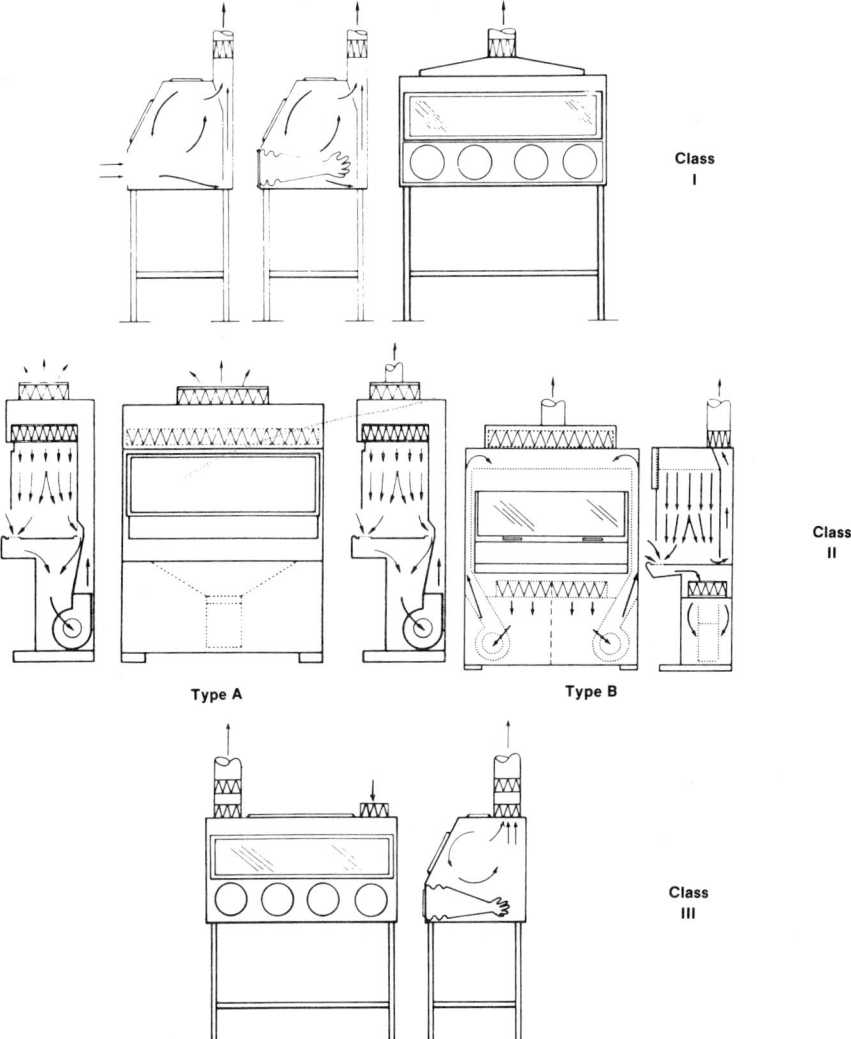

Fig. 6-8. Diagrams of the three classes of biological safety cabinets.

cabinets. Fans should be turned on when a cabinet is in use to assure proper air flow and should be left on for one-half hour after the work is completed. Safety centrifuges and shaking machines should be housed in ventilated safety cabinets. When these are in use, the glove panels should be closed. When equipment used in a biological safety cabinet is removed, it must be autoclaved or disinfected. Biosafety cabinets are *not* to be substituted for *any* other type of hood or ventilation.

The National Institutes of Health (NIH) recommends that all biohazardous materials be manipulated in a suitable, ventilated biosafety cabinet. Examples suggested by NIH include opening of test tubes, flasks, and bottles, grinding of tissues, blending of cultures, and opening of lyophilized tubes.

Class I Safety Cabinet

Class I safety cabinets are ventilated cabinets for minimal personnel protection, having an open front with an inward flow of air away from the operator (Fig. 6-9). This provides negative pressure with

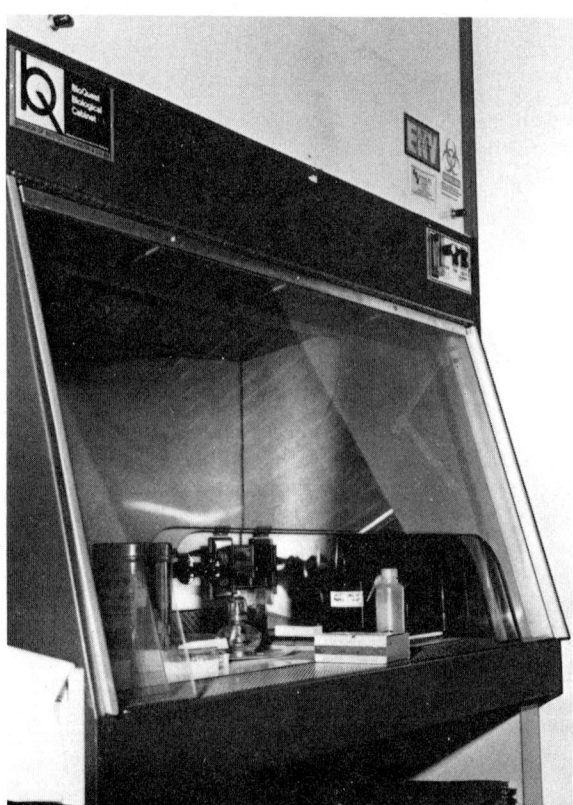

Fig. 6-9. A well-ordered biological safety cabinet. When materials normally kept inside are moved from the cabinet, they *must* be disinfected.

respect to the laboratory in general. In operation, 50 linear ft/min to 75 linear ft/min of air should cross the frontal opening. Air is exhausted through a high-efficiency particulate air (HEPA) filter which has a particle-removal efficiency of no less than 99.97% for 0.3 μm particles. Class I cabinets can be used for work with low- to moderate-risk agents when no product protection is required.

Class II Safety Cabinet

Class II safety cabinets are open-front cabinets for personnel and work protection. They utilize mass recirculated air flow and have HEPA-filtered exhaust and HEPA-filtered recirculated air. They can be used for work with low- to moderate-risk agents and must never be used with explosives, radioisotopes, toxics, or flammable chemicals. With each pass of air, this cabinet recirculates 80% to 90% of air through HEPA filters and draws in 10% to 20% new air.

Class III Safety Cabinet

Class III safety cabinets are not found or required in the clinical laboratory and are not discussed further. They are used when maximum containment is necessary, as is often the case in research laboratories doing viral or tumor research.

Classification of Etiologic Agents on the Basis of Hazard

The Classification of Etiologic Agents on the Basis of Hazard is presented to provide the technologist with a relative measure of hazard of the infectious agents that may be encountered in the laboratory.* This classification system includes bacteria, fungi, *Rickettsia, Chlamydia,*

---

*The listing given here is adapted from U.S. Department of Health, Education and Welfare, Centers for Disease Control: Classification of Etiologic Agents on the Basis of Hazard, 1976. In 1984, a joint CDC/NIH publication, Biosafety in Microbiological and Biomedical Laboratories, will replace Classification of Etiologic Agents on the Basis of Hazard (1976) and the Proposed Biosafety Guidelines for Microbiological and Biomedical Laboratories (unpublished). These new guidelines do not substantially change the recommended safety levels presented here. They generally update and reorganize the contents of the previous publications and provide the reader with exact precautions and safety levels for each named organism. The booklet will be available from the Office of Biosafety, Centers for Disease Control, Atlanta GA 30333.

and parasites. The levels of protective biosafety required in hospitals, schools, and research laboratories are based on this system, which considers the etiologic agents that are to be expected in each situation. The lower the classification number, the lower the hazard of the organism. The basis for classification follows:

- Class I—Organisms listed here are relatively or completely nonpathogenic under ordinary conditions and require no special apparatus to handle. Organisms not specifically listed in other categories are included here.
- Class II—Organisms listed here are agents of ordinary potential hazard. This class includes agents that may produce disease of varying degrees of severity but that are contained by ordinary laboratory techniques. (This includes routine clinical-laboratory organisms.)
- Class III—Organisms listed here are agents involving special hazard and include pathogens that require special conditions for containment (*e.g.,* TB and *Brucella*).
- Class IV—Organisms listed here are agents that require the most stringent conditions for their containment because they are extremely hazardous to laboratory personnel or may cause serious epidemic disease.

Agents of Disinfection, Sterilization, Antisepsis

An overview of the major agents of disinfection, sterilization, and antisepsis is provided in Table 6-6. It illustrates the wide variety of chemical and physical agents available and gives some idea of their relative usefulness. Disinfection, sterilization, and antisepsis are of utmost importance in the microbiology laboratory not only for the safety and well-being of the laboratory staff, but for housekeeping personnel, patients, and the surrounding community as well. (Commercial names of the agents are given in Table 6-7.)

The best overall method to achieve sterility in the clinical laboratory is to autoclave. Even with autoclaving, however, care must be taken to assure proper temperature, proper pressure, and steam penetration to the center of the object being sterilized; otherwise, the desired effect will not be obtained. Other methods of sterilization, disinfection, and antisepsis must be routinely used, however, because of the nature or size of the objects that are contaminated. For example, ground-glass connections may be affected by autoclaving, and a highly contaminated cabinet cannot physically fit into an autoclave. Other methods have their specific advantages and limitations, but among considerations in choosing the treatment for contaminated equipment, supplies, and surfaces are the following:

Type and volume of waste or material to be decontaminated (*e.g.,* culture media, contaminated waste, water bath)
Contact time needed
Required concentration of agent
Toxicity of agents to personnel using it or residual toxicity on item decontaminated
Degree of contamination
Amount of protein or organic material on item to be decontaminated

Useful Definitions for Sterilization and Decontamination Agents

- Antiseptic or bacteriostatic—inhibits the growth of organisms, but does not necessarily kill them
- Aseptic—procedure conducted in a manner that prevents the introduction of septic material
- Bactericide—germicide; kills vegetative bacteria
- Decontaminate—to eliminate danger of infection for unprotected persons.
- Disinfection—the killing of infectious agents
- Etiologic agent—organism or toxin that may cause human disease
- High-efficiency particulate air (HEPA) filter—a disposable, extended medium, dry-type filter with a particle-removal efficiency of no less than 99.9% for 0.3 μm particles
- Infectious—capable of causing disease in a susceptible host
- Sterilization—the complete elimination of viable microorganisms
- Viable—able to grow and multiply; viability of microbial cells is often dependent on a precise set of culture conditions

Table 6-6. Agents of Disinfection, Sterilization, and Antisepsis

TYPE	COMMENTS
Physical	
Radiation	
• Ultraviolet (UV)	Direct exposure is necessary because a protein coat or dirt can prevent penetration of microbe. UV bulbs must be cleaned often. UV presents eye-burn hazard.
Temperature	Heat sterilization, especially with moist heat, is best agent overall
• Pasteurization	Dry-heat hot-air oven, 160° for 1 hour good for glassware; most other items 2–4 hr.
• Dry heat—hot-air oven, red-heat flame	Needs longer time, higher temperature than autoclave.
• Wet heat—autoclave	Most reliable agent. Must be routinely checked with spore strips. All biohazardous waste should be autoclaved in special bags before further disposal. All air must be replaced by steam. Required heat level must get to center of load.
• Freezing • Incineration	Combustion yields gas and ash for landfill.
Mechanical	
• Sonic and ultrasonic waves	
• Filtration	
• Membranes	

(continues)

Table 6-6. Agents of Disinfection, Sterilization, and Antisepsis (continued)

TYPE	COMMENTS
Chemical	
	Chemicals are not as good as sterilization by moist heat, but obviously they are the only agents that can be used in spills, wiping the outsides of specimen tubes, etc.
	Most are toxic or irritating to user and reactions must be noted.
Phenols	Denature proteins; some residual activity; organics don't interfere
• Phenol—1%–3% of 5%–10% concentrate	Moderately effective
• Tricresol	Mix with soap
• Hexylresorcinol	Good skin disinfectant, low level of activity for contaminated surfaces
• Hexachlorophene 1%–3%	Good skin disinfectant, low level of activity for contaminated surfaces
Halogens	
• Iodine—tincture of iodine (2%–7% iodine in 70% aqueous ethyl alcohol), KI added	
• Iodophor—iodine complexed to a detergent (*e.g.*, Wescodyne)	This is only fairly effective; takes longer to penetrate virus or protein coat. Iodophors have residual action; relatively nontoxic
• Chlorine—200–2000 ppm available chlorine	Chlorine is neutralized by organic materials
• Hypochlorite—5% sodium hypochlorite	Considered best agent against hepatitis virus
Heavy metals—mercurials 1:1000–1:500	Very unsatisfactory
Alcohols (disinfectants & antiseptics)	Denature proteins; skin disinfectant

(continues)

Table 6-6. Agents of Disinfection, Sterilization, and Antisepsis (continued)

TYPE	COMMENTS
• Ethyl alcohol 70%–90%	Fairly effective; no residual action
• 50% glycerol	Preservative properties
• Isopropanol 70%–90%	Fair
Oxidants	
• Hydrogen peroxide	
• Peracetic acid	
Alkylating agents	
• Formaldehyde 3%–8% in H$_2$O	Intermediate level of activity
• Formaldehyde 8% in alcohol	High level of activity; kills vegetative bacteria, spores, viruses, often chemical of choice
• Glutaraldehyde 2%	High level of activity
• Gas/vapor—ethylene oxide or formaldehyde gas	Used for slow sterilization of supplies that are unstable with heat; both may be dangerous to exposed personnel. Marketed as nonflammable in freon or CO$_2$ mixture. Items should not come into direct contact with human skin until 24 hr after gas sterilization.
Synthetic detergents	Cationic best at high pH; anionic best at low pH
• Cationic—quaternary ammonium 1:750–1:500	Low level of activity
• Anionic	Low level of activity

Table 6-7. Commercial Names of Commonly Used Disinfectants

QUATERNARY AMMO-NIUM COMPOUNDS	PHENOLIC COMPOUNDS	CHLORINE COMPOUNDS	IODOPHOR	FORMALDEHYDE	GLUTARALDEHYDE
A-33	Hil-Phene	Chloramine-T	Hy-Sine	Sterac	Cidex
CDQ	Matar	Clorox	Ioprep		
End-Bac	Mikro-Bac	Purex	Mikroklene		
Hi-Tor	O-Syl		Wescodyne		
Mikro-Quat					

(Acapted from U.S. Environmental Protection Agency: Draft Manual for Infectious Waste Management, pp. 4-36, 1982)

7

Fire, Electricity, and Compressed Gases

This chapter addresses three important safety hazards: fire, electricity, and compressed gases. They have been separated from other chapters' discussions of hazards related to specific laboratories because they may be encountered anywhere in the clinical laboratory. Gas cylinders of varying sizes and contents can be found in microbiology as well as in chemistry. Electric outlets are ubiquitous and so are electronic instruments. Fire prevention is mandatory in storage areas as well as at each workbench. It is essential, therefore, that each laboratory worker pay serious attention to these hazards and acquire a healthy respect for them.

Although no explicit discussion is provided of the potential cause-and-effect relationships among these three types of hazard such relationships should be apparent to the thoughtful reader. Safety precautions for each of these three hazards include reference to or consideration of the other two.

FIRE

Fire is a complicated phenomenon that is often not well understood. It may be defined generally as the rapid oxidation of a fuel by an oxidizer in the presence of an ignition source resulting in the liberation of heat and light. The minimum temperature to which the substance (in air) must be heated in order to initiate or cause self-sustained combustion, independently of the heating or heated element, is the *ignition temperature.* As the temperature increases, there is an increase in the number of molecules that are thermally activated until a threshold is reached. At this point the reaction becomes self-sustaining until fuel or oxygen or both have been consumed. Whether the combustible material is solid, liquid, or gas, initiation of the flame reaction always occurs in the gas or vapor phase.

A fuel, an oxidizing agent, and an ignition source must *always* be present for combustion to occur. These are often referred to as the *fire triangle.* Fuels include materials *not* already in their most oxidized state (any material consisting primarily of carbon and hydrogen can be oxidized). Oxygen is the most common oxidizing agent and can be provided by air or chemicals that release oxygen (*e.g.,* sodium nitrate).

Explosions differ from fire or combustion. An explosion is an effect produced by the sudden violent expansion of gases. Explosions result from chemical, physical, mechanical, or atomic changes. Fire- and explosion-prevention measures for flammable and combustible liquids include one or more of the following: exclusion of sources of ignition (*e.g.,* smoking), exclusion of air (*i.e.,* smothering), storage of flammable and combustible liquids in closed containers, and prevention of vapor accumulation by ventilation or provision of an inert-gas atmosphere. Extinguishing methods for fires caused by flammable liquids include stoppage of the fuel supply, exclusion of air, and cooling of the liquid.

Fires can kill in a variety of ways. Among them are production of carbon monoxide, toxic fumes, and intense heat and depletion of oxygen. The most frequent causes of laboratory fires are carelessness, inattention, lack of knowledge, smoking, unattended operations, unsafe environments, faulty electricity (*e.g.,* bad wiring), sparks from electrical apparatus, fires in fume hoods, and circuit overloads.

Classification of Fires and Extinguishers

Fires and extinguishers are classified into groups according to the nature of the combustible material (Fig. 7-1):

1. **Class A**
   Fires
   - Ordinary combustible materials such as wood, papers, towels, and laboratory coats; elements that require the quenching and cooling action of water or water-based solutions for extinguishment
   Extinguishers
   - Foam
   - Loaded stream
   - Multipurpose dry chemical
2. **Class B**
   Fires
   - Flammable liquids and gases, oil, paint, grease; elements that require the blockage of oxygen from the fuel for extinguishment
   Extinguishers
   - Bromotrifluoromethane (HALON 1301)
   - Bromochlorodifluoromethane (HALON 1211)
   - Carbon dioxide
   - Dry chemical (sodium- or potassium-bicarbonate or potassium-chloride based)
   - Foam
   - Loaded stream
3. **Class C**
   Fires
   - Energized (live) electrical equipment; require nonconductive media for extinguishment (foam, water, and water-type extinguishers can conduct electricity back to the extinguisher and kill the operator)
   Extinguishers
   - HALON 1301
   - HALON 1211
   - Carbon dioxide

- Dry chemical
- For deenergized (current-off) electrical-equipment fires, Class A or B extinguishers may be used. For Class C fires, cut off electrical power if possible. ABC-type dry-chemical fire extinguishers can be used for Class A, B, and C fires.

4. *Class D*
   Fires
   - Combustible and reactive metals such as sodium, potassium, magnesium, and lithium; the most difficult fires to control and extinguish; spread and explosion occur easily.

   Extinguishers
   - Sand (Fig. 7-2)
   - Dry-powder media applied by scoop
   - *Never* use wet extinguishing agents

5. *Class E*
   Fires
   - *Cannot* be put out and must be allowed to burn; fire departments usually evacuate under these conditions and try to protect surrounding structures.

Fire extinguishers have a limited range and length of time of operation. The letter on each is for the appropriate class of fire; the number on each refers to its relative extinguishing potential. Extinguishers should be placed and distributed according to the hazards present. The amount of extinguishing agent should be proportionate to the combustibility and amount of reactive materials in use. There should be one extinguisher per workbench. It should be a convenient size, up to 10-pound charge, for ease of handling. In addition, each laboratory should have a backup extinguisher of the dry-chemical powder type.

Extinguishers themselves, as well as toxic combustion products, may present health hazards. For this reason, some extinguishing agents are limited by law (*e.g.,* carbon-tetrachloride and inversion extinguishers may *not* be used). The sulfuric acid in soda-ash extinguishers presents a serious burn hazard and these extinguishers should be avoided. Other considerations include damage to equipment and the residual effects of extinguishing materials. For minimizing damage to computers, sprinklers and carbon-dioxide or HALON 1301 extinguishers are best.

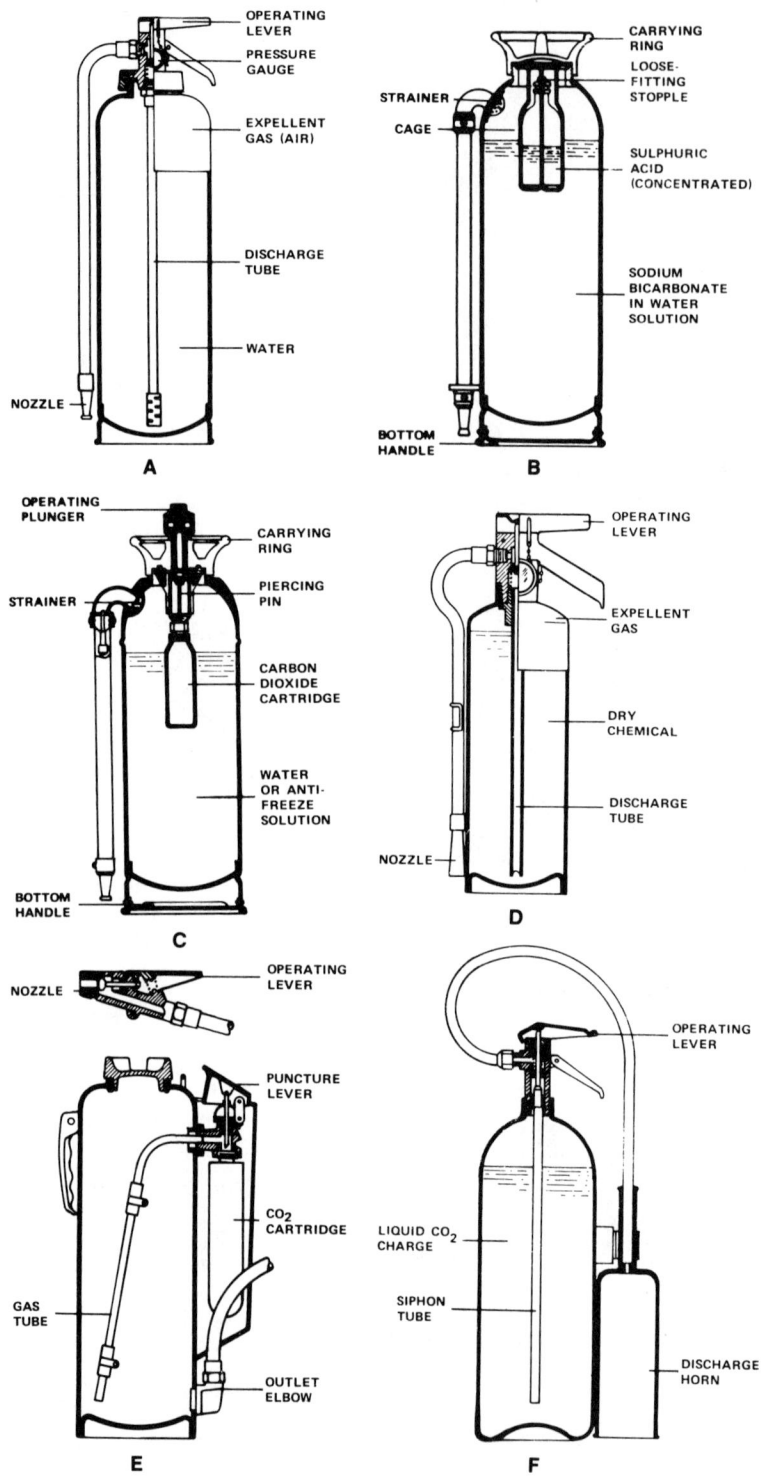

A

- OPERATING LEVER
- PRESSURE GAUGE
- EXPELLENT GAS (AIR)
- DISCHARGE TUBE
- WATER
- NOZZLE

B

- CARRYING RING
- LOOSE-FITTING STOPPLE
- STRAINER
- CAGE
- SULPHURIC ACID (CONCENTRATED)
- SODIUM BICARBONATE IN WATER SOLUTION
- BOTTOM HANDLE

C

- OPERATING PLUNGER
- CARRYING RING
- PIERCING PIN
- STRAINER
- CARBON DIOXIDE CARTRIDGE
- WATER OR ANTI-FREEZE SOLUTION
- BOTTOM HANDLE

D

- OPERATING LEVER
- EXPELLENT GAS
- DRY CHEMICAL
- DISCHARGE TUBE
- NOZZLE

E

- NOZZLE
- OPERATING LEVER
- PUNCTURE LEVER
- CO$_2$ CARTRIDGE
- GAS TUBE
- OUTLET ELBOW

F

- OPERATING LEVER
- LIQUID CO$_2$ CHARGE
- SIPHON TUBE
- DISCHARGE HORN

Fire Safety Program

Laboratories are required by law to have fire-resistant structures, designed with safety in mind, and the presence of fire-fighting and safety equipment. It is necessary, however, to enhance these required features with safe working practices, fire-fighting training, and knowledge of fire hazards. These should be incorporated into the mandatory fire safety program, which requires good laboratory management and employee cooperation for success. Training and drills are an essential part of this program and local fire departments often gladly aid in conducting training exercises for laboratory staff members.

A self-inspection fire-safety checklist that includes at least the following items should be part of the fire safety plan:

A posted fire plan
A posted and enforced smoking policy
Fire extinguishers—correct type, properly maintained, well placed, and adequate number
Exits—marked, with clear passage, doors unlocked
Flammable liquids—correct quantities, properly stored, used, and disposed
Storeroom—inventoried, with clear aisles, incompatibles separated (Fig. 7-3)
Heating devices—approved type, properly used
Fire detection—correct type, properly maintained, well placed
Fire doors—correct type, operable, unblocked
Fire separations—without openings or violations
Refrigerators—clearly marked for type of storage
Flammable-liquid storage cabinets—correct quantities, contents, construction, ventilation
Smoke separations—without openings in walls operable doors

Checklists from insurance companies and the College of American Pathologists provide an inspection format for the entire laboratory.

◀Fig. 7-1. Types of fire extinguishers include (A) Stored-pressure water extinguisher, used for Class A fires; (B) soda acid extinguisher, used for Class A fires; (C) gas-cartridge water extinguisher, used for Class A fires; (D) stored-pressure dry chemical hand-portable extinguisher, used for Class A, B, and C fires; (E) dry chemical cartridge-operated extinguisher, used for Class A, B, C, and D fires; and (F) carbon-dioxide extinguisher, used for Class B and C fires.

Reporting of laboratory fires to the National Fire Protection Association (NFPA) is not mandatory; however, in an NFPA survey of serious hospital fires that were reported in 1970, out of 381 fires, 27 originated in laboratories. By comparison, 28 were in storerooms, 63 in patients' rooms, and 25 in operating rooms (Tables 7-1, 7-2).

Good Laboratory Practices for Fire Prevention and Control

- Assign individual responsibilities for actions to be taken in the event of a fire (*e.g.,* call fire department, turn off main switches, order evacuation of staff).
- Continuously enforce general fire-safety concerns.
- Remember that good laboratory and workbench housekeeping are mandatory (*e.g.,* adequate trash removal, safe handling of cleaning materials, limitation of chemicals at hand to day's needs)
- Remember that there is absolutely *no* smoking in the laboratory except in designated areas.

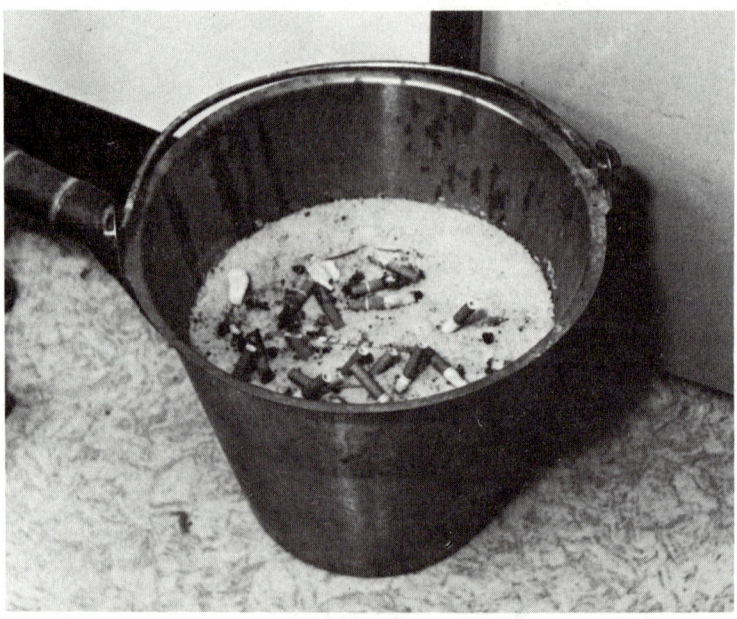

Fig. 7-2. Sand buckets must be available in the laboratory for extinguishing fires; they are not for extinguishing cigarettes. This figure represents a violation of the fire code.

- Follow electrical safety precautions (*e.g.,* only UL-approved equipment in use, equipment disconnected after use).
- Use only approved extension cords, and then as just a temporary measure. The safest policy is to use *no* extension cords.
- Handle and store flammable liquids as fire laws require (*e.g.,* approved containers, limited amounts, specified sizes of fire cabinets).
- Keep storage areas neat and inventoried. Store incompatible chemicals separately.
- Keep exits well marked and obstruction free.

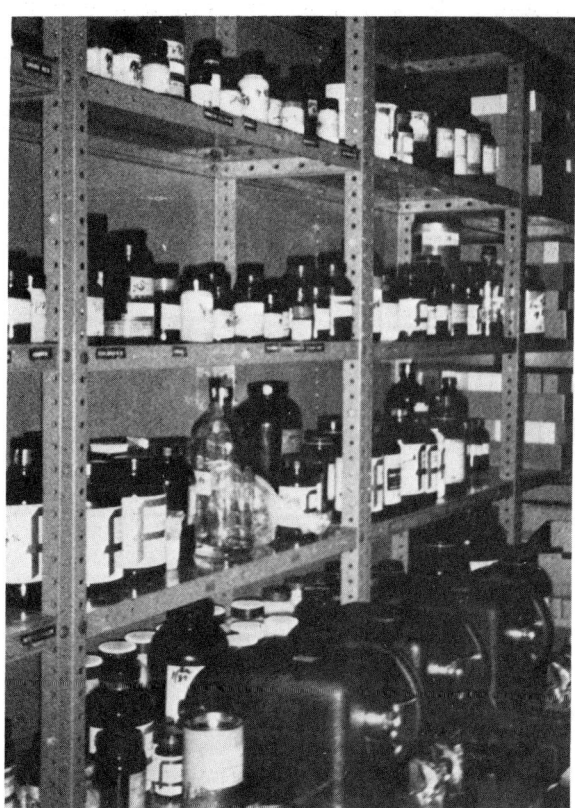

Fig. 7-3. This storeroom is cluttered and poorly organized. Shelves have no guardrails and the chemicals can be easily knocked over. There is no way to inventory the chemicals in this storeroom or to remove outdated ones.

Table 7-1. Typical Fuel-Load Occupancies

LOAD	PLACE
Light	Office with metal furnishings
	File rooms (metal files)
	Classrooms
	Hospitals' patient areas
	Dining rooms
	Conference rooms, auditoriums
	Restrooms, locker rooms (metal lockers)
Moderate	Department-store sales areas
	Most storerooms
	Library stacks
	Rooms with paper or records on open shelves
	Most industrial operations
	Drafting rooms, mapmaking rooms
	Offices with wooden furnishings
	Shops—no flammable liquids or production woodworking
High	Flammable liquid operations
	Woodworking shops
	Places with oils
	Places with explosives and pyrotechnics
	Trash rooms
	General storage warehouses
	Chemical or other laboratories involving flammable liquids

Nelson HE: *J Am Soc Saf Eng.,* 10, 17, 1965. Used with permission.

- Keep fire doors closed.
- Use and store compressed gases only as safety rules permit.
- Develop and rehearse an evacuation plan.
- Make sure fire detectors, alarms, and extinguishers are properly located, well marked, well maintained (once yearly) and inspected (monthly) for good working order (Fig.7-4). They must be replaced after being discharged or when being repaired.
- Tag each extinguisher with maintenance schedule and inspector's

initials. Permanently mount extinguishers at the approved height.

- Keep safety cabinets and safety cans available and use them properly.
- Keep powder extinguishers or drums full at all times.
- Keep personal protective equipment available, sanitary, reliable, and appropriate to the hazards present (*e.g.*, eye, hand, face, or head protectors; respirators).

Fire Handling

If a fire starts, act quickly (Tables 7-1 and 7-2). One person should ring the alarm while another begins fighting the fire. If there is a person (or his clothing) on fire, he should be wrapped in a fire blanket or drenched under the emergency shower. Rescue injured persons first. A

(Text continues on p. 200)

Table 7-2. Fire-Department Response to Hospital Alarms*

MATERIAL OR HAZARD INVOLVED	NUMBER OF FIRES
Sheets, bedclothes, linens, pillows, gowns, etc. (all articles where patient carelessness was possible cause)	574 (42%)
Ashtrays, trash containers, wastebaskets, burns on tables, overstuffed chairs, etc. (all articles where patient, visitor, or employee carelessness was possible cause)	326 (23%)
Electric motors, malfunctioning laundry equipment, light fixtures, laboratory and x-ray equipment, etc. (all tools and equipment that would be the responsibility of the hospital)	285 (21%)
Smoke conditions (visible smoke and odors of possible smoke)	111 (8%)
False alarms (faulty alarm systems or false calls to hospitals)	87 (6%)

*13 hospitals—4680 beds; 4-year study (1966–1969) (Minneapolis Bureau of Fire Prevention, Education Division). Used with permission.

EXAMPLES OF LABORATORY FIRES

Descriptions of a few laboratory fires are included in NFPA FR 61-1, "Occupancy Fire Record Hospitals." Some laboratory fires and explosions are described below:

Tissue-Processor Fire Operated 24 hours per day, but unattended from 11 PM to 7 AM, a tissue processor was suspected of causing $200,000 damage because the incident occurred after 11 P.M. and there were no detectors or automatic extinguishing equipment in the laboratory. Flammable liquids in glass containers stored in an open shell below the equipment contributed to the intensity of the fire.

Aside from damage to the laboratory, electrical cables in the corridor near the incident shorted and caused power to be interrupted in the hospital. Fire doors closed, but the fire alarm was not sounded.

"Walking" Motor Fire A motor, which had been connected to inadequately secured apparatus, "walked" off a bench and caught fire.

Incinerator's Explosion The operators received minor burns as they dumped contents of GI cans into a top feed incinerator, detonations were caused by "empty" ether cans.

Perchloric Acid Explosion A maintenance worker was killed by an explosion resulting from the prodding of the cover plate of a fan which had been routinely exhausting perchloric acid fumes.

Cellulose Nitrate Centrifuge Tubes A technician suffered severe injuries when an explosion blew the door from a steam autoclave which had been sterilizing blood samples contained in cellulose nitrate tubes. In a different instance, cellulose nitrate culture tubes were destroyed by fire while within the closed compartment.

A technician noticed nitrogen oxide fumes seeping from the oven which was drying cellulose-nitrate tubes. Upon opening the door to inspect, a mild explosion occurred followed by the tubes bursting into flames. A new employee had assumed that the oven-control dial read in centrigrade when actually it was marked with an arbitrary graduation. The damage was slight but the potential was reminiscent of the 1929 Cleveland Clinic X-ray film fire, which killed 125 people.

Explosion Hazard of Scintillation Counters In a refrigerated scintillation counter, enough solvent vapor may penetrate through plastic bottles or leak from plastic snap-type caps to form an explosive concentration in the box. Many organics penetrate at varying rates through some plastics.

Hot-Plate Fires Acetone, being poured at the sink in a patient treatment lab, was ignited by a nearby hot plate which had just been turned off. The technician dropped the container, which was metal and which, fortunately, fell in an upright position. The patient was safely evacuated but the fire was intense enough to melt the sweated water pipefittings of the window ventilator.

Petroleum ether caught fire while a chemist was pouring it in a fume hood from its large glass container—presumably ignited by a nearby hot plate, which had recently been turned off. He dropped the glass container on the floor and ran from the room. The bottle broke; ignition caused enough pressure to blow open the lab escape hatch and slam the entrance door shut.

Refrigerator Explosion 80 ml of diazomethane dissolved in ether detonated in a domestic-type refrigerator. The door blew open, the frame bowed out, and the plastic lining ignited, causing a heavy blanket of soot to be deposited far down the adjoining corridor.

Pressure-Filter Fire At an eastern hospital pharmacy, a fire-conscious technician prepared for pressure filtering of 50 gal of isopropyl alcohol by placing a towel on a table adjacent to the pump; in the event of fire he planned to smother flames of alcohol inadvertently spilled on his person. As he attempted to turn on the pump, he reached for the towel as he had previously rehearsed in his mind but, in doing so, he tripped over the hose which was conducting alcohol by gravity from a large open kettle to the suction side of the pump. The hose slipped from its fittings thereby dumping 50 gal of the flaming solvent onto the floor. He escaped with minor injuries but the pharmacy was destroyed.

(Many fires are intensified by an unfortunate sequence of minor unsafe practices which in themselves seem almost too insignificant to worry about.)

Ampoules Explode An ampoule of tissue exploded like a firecracker moments after being removed from a liquid nitrogen refrigerator. The legs of the female assistant were peppered with powdered glass. Such an explosion occurs as a result of liquid nitrogen being drawn into an imperfectly sealed ampoule through pinhole imperfections. As the ampoule is removed from the bath room temperature expands the entrapped nitrogen rapidly, causing it to burst with much violence.

(continued)

Chromatography Fire Hazard Chromatography apparatus operating through the night had collected 2,500 ml of cyclohexane, with 200 ml remaining in the solvent reservoir when two explosions occurred. Ignition was attributed to sparks from electrical controls on the sampling device. (Based on DuPont Safety News of May 24, 1965.)

Water Bath Fire When the thermostat on a water bath malfunctioned, the bath overheated, causing the acrylic lid to sag and contact the heater elements. A fire resulted. Heater equipment should always be protected by over-temperature shutoffs. (Based on DuPont Safety News, June 14, 1965.)

Cyclopropane Explosion Upon opening the valve of a cylinder supposedly containing only cyclopropane, the cylinder exploded with extensive fragmentation, killing six and mutilating three others. This occurred in a Chilean hospital operating room in 1964.

The cylinder had been partially filled in error, by oxygen and subsequently charged with cyclopropane. The valve, regulator and fittings were unsuitable for oxygen, thus providing the conditions for a classical organic-oxidizer explosion. (From NPFA Quarterly, 1/64, 222.)

Centrifuge Fire A small centrifuge, being used under a lab hood to separate a flammable hydrocarbon slurry, flashed in the operator's face. The motor was nonexplosionproof; the exhaust fan had been turned off.

Peroxide Explosion A distillation apparatus exploded within a lab fume hood. It was caused by the detonation of the residual peroxide. The drawn sash prevented injury, although the electric mantle was torn to shreds. The investigator was using "some isopropyl ether" which had been kept in a clear glass bottle. He allowed the distillation to continue to dryness.

Investigators should become more aware of the nature of

ether peroxide formations. Dioxane and ethyl and isopropyl ethers are the most common offenders. Age, sunlight, air space above liquid, and clear glass containers help to create explosive peroxides. Test frequently for peroxide; filter out peroxides through a column of 80 mesh Alorco activated alumina, as suggested by Dasler & Baure, Ind. Eng. Chem. Anal, Ed. 18.52 (1964). Never leave distillations unattended.

Spinning Gas Cylinder While a large uncapped gas cylinder was being loaded on a freight elevator prior to laboratory delivery, it fell over. The valve opened slightly on the floor. A quick thinking attendant shut off the valve before damaging momentum could be attained. Moving an uncapped cylinder within a limited area is permissible provided it is strapped to a carrying cart.

Steam-Bath Flush Flammable vapors from a batch of solvent which had been poured into a drain upstairs floated into the chamber of a steam bath fixture. As the investigator lit a Bunsen burner adjacent to the steam bath, the flammable vapors ignited, causing a quick hot flash. The rubber tubing was burned beyond recognition. The hood sash protected the investigator's face so he escaped with no injury other than singed eyebrows. ROOM OCCUPANTS SHOULD RUN WATER INTO UNUSED STEAM-BATH TRAPS AND ALL OTHER UNUSED TRAPS ABOUT TWICE A MONTH.

Fume Hood Operations About an hour after the electrical system failed because of a substation fire, toxic gases began to permeate through portions of the hospital.

Closing down the electric system, either accidentally or announced, cuts off all hood and room ventilation and lack of ventilation may lead to sudden contamination of large areas. Upon announcement that the electrical system has failed, or is about to be shut down, experimental processes which produce hazardous exhaust should be slowed down or stopped.

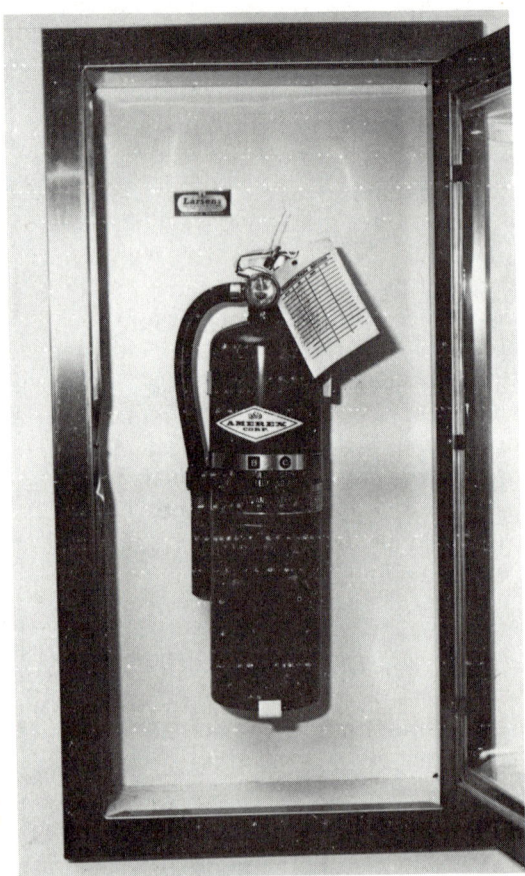

Fig. 7-4. Fire extinguishers must be easily accessible, appropriate for the materials in use, and lightweight. Note maintenance tags for inspection records.

small fire should be put out quickly by laboratory personnel, but only if this can be done safely. (Large fires should be left to professionals and laboratory staff should be evacuated.) Respirators should be worn if toxic fumes may be present. Inform firemen as to what chemicals are involved or may become involved. Both CO_2 and water extinguishers should be directed toward the base of the flames, then onto the smoldering material to cool it off. For flammable liquids, sweep the flame off the burning surface with the extinguisher. Direct dry-chemical extinguishers toward the base of the fire and quickly sweep them from side to side, being careful to prevent splashing.

ELECTRICITY

Electricity presents a significant human health hazard because the human body is a ready conductor of electric current. This "stream of moving electrons" (current) produces the deleterious health effects that result in burns or life-threatening disruption of the central nervous system. For this reason, the extensive use of electric instruments in the laboratory must be approached by the laboratory professional with both knowledge and caution.

It is an implicit assumption in this section on electricity that all electric equipment being used in the laboratory is approved for electric safety by Underwriters Laboratory (UL) or an equivalent body. Faulty equipment, homemade equipment, and temporary electric repairs are unacceptable and they will not be considered here.

Various standard-setting and testing bodies (*e.g.,* UL, NFPA), after much research into the safe use of electricity, have developed electric and fire codes and standards that minimize both hazards. Universal color coding for wiring carrying electricity is an example of this safety effort. "Hot wires" have gray or black insulation; common wires, white insulation; and ground wires, green or yellow insulation. The color coding is intended to prevent improper electric connections and to provide visual reinforcement for proper connections.

All electric installations and equipment in the laboratory must be in compliance with the National Electrical Code, NFPA 70-1971, and American National Standards Institute 01-1971. Mandatory grounding of equipment and circuits, unobstructed switchgear and panel boards and mandatory covers over electric outlets are included in these codes.

In laboratories where volatile flammables are used, the electric equipment used must be of the nonsparking type. This must be kept in mind when temporary electric equipment (*e.g.,* vacuum cleaners, electric drills) is brought into these laboratories.

Another requirement in the clinical laboratory is the grounding of all electric equipment and outlets. Although most equipment now comes equipped with three-pronged plugs, which ground the instrument and polarize the connection, sometimes it may be necessary to use a substitute ground connector or "pigtail," which *must* be connected before turning on the equipment (Fig. 7-5). Its use prevents an unplanned electric current from being routed through the person using the equipment. Instruments must be tested by a qualified electrician

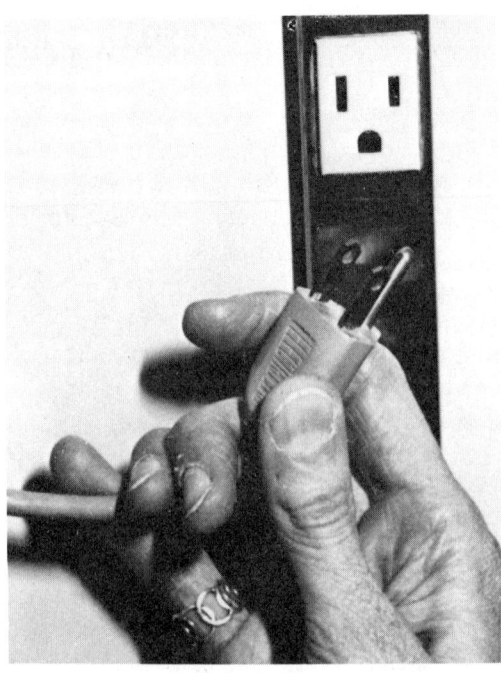

Fig. 7-5. All electric appliances in the laboratory must be grounded with a three-pronged plug. An adapter is acceptable in some situations.

to assure proper functioning before they are put into routine use. Additionally, electric repairs should be made only by qualified personnel.

Safety Procedures for Using Electricity (Fig. 7-6)

- In case of electric shock, turn off power at the source or separate the victim from the source *with a nonconductor*. Provide mouth-to-mouth resuscitation if needed.
- If fire results, quickly turn off electricity *at the source*.
- Remember that a master switch to cut off electricity to all stations is desirable for all laboratory AC equipment.
- Make sure that all electric equipment shows listing and approval by UL or a similar body.
- Make sure that all electric appliances and equipment are grounded in accordance with the National Electric Code.
- Have all "homemade" electric apparatus inspected and approved by a competent electrician.
- Remember that electric equipment can be altered by a competent electrician to make it safe in hazardous or flammable atmospheres (*e.g.,* switches, lights, motors, and electric contacts are removed to remote or purged locations).

- Never overload electric circuits.
- Make sure that all technicians know where electric controls (*e.g.,* panel box) are located.
- Periodically check all wiring circuits, grounds, insulation, and so on for worn, frayed, or loose connections.
- Immediately disconnect equipment producing a "tingle" and do not use it until it is repaired.
- Make sure that extension cords are short, of proper size and type, and used for no more than 24 hours. Some hospitals do not allow their use at all. "Hard-wire" them in and carefully place them to avoid causing a physical hazard.
- Do not work on electric devices when the power is on.
- Treat all electric devices as if they are live.
- Enclose all electric contacts and conductors.
- Carefully choose cleaning solvents for electric equipment with

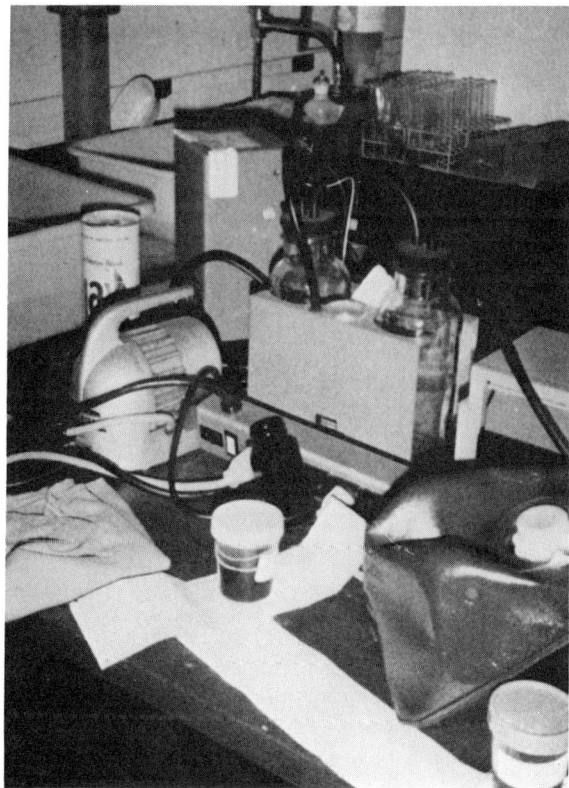

Fig. 7-6. The careless use of materials and specimens represented here creates obvious hazards, including electric and infection hazards.

respect to toxicity, flammability, and potential damage to the equipment. Follow manufacturers' instructions for all equipment used.

- Never handle electric equipment with wet hands, feet, or body or when standing on a wet floor.
- When electric equipment must be touched, use the back of the hand; otherwise, when shock occurs, the muscle contraction "freezes" the hand to the conductor.
- Avoid storing highly flammable liquids near electric equipment (Fig. 7-7).

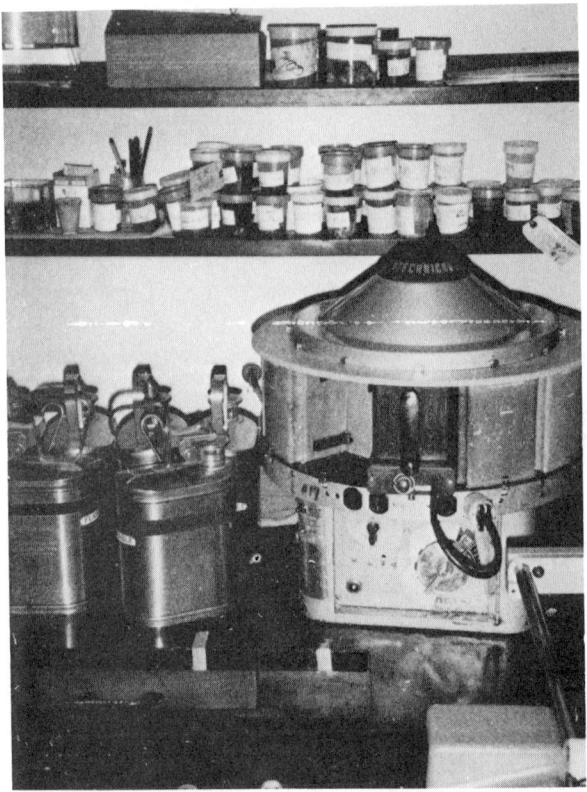

Fig. 7-7. Multiple hazards are present when equipment, flammables, and specimens are stored in this manner. The presence of safety cans among the flammables and clutter should not reassure anyone.

- Never cut off the "ground" and never remove green pigtail.
- Water and gas pipes are grounded. Never touch a water or gas pipe and an electric current simultaneously.
- Immediately replace worn insulation and wires.
- If liquid spills on an electric motor, turn the motor off, dry it well, and caution others against its use.
- Remember that radios, fans, and so on, if allowed in the laboratory, must also be grounded.
- Leave a clear, unobstructed path to the breaker box.

COMPRESSED GASES

Because of the pressure required to maintain them and the apparatus and conditions surrounding their use, compressed gases present an unusual and serious hazard whenever they are used. Personnel in each laboratory should be familiar with approved procedures for the use of compressed gases and should not be misled by the seemingly indestructible construction of the cylinders. Rules pertaining to the safe use, storage, and transport of compressed gases must be followed exactly and at all times. The most vulnerable part of a compressed-gas cylinder is the main valve stem. If this is accidentally sheared, the resulting "torpedo" cannot easily be controlled or corrected. In addition, the use of some compressed gases may present the hazards of toxicity, flammability, and explosion as well as of pressure.

Compressed gases are used in many of the clinical laboratories and are found in varying sizes and in pure or mixed states. These gases are defined by the Department of Transportation as "any material or mixture having in the container either an absolute pressure exceeding 40 pounds per square inch at 70°F, or an absolute pressure exceeding 104 pounds per square inch at 130° or both; or any liquid flammable material having a Reid vapor pressure exceeding 40 pounds per square inch at 100°F."

Compressed gases are more hazardous than are liquid and solid materials because of their unique properties: pressure, diffuseness, low flash points (if flammable), low boiling points, and often no detectability by vision or odor. All rules and regulations are, therefore, designed to contain the materials and to properly control pressure and flow.

Cylinder Information

- Do not accept cylinders with physical distortions.
- Do not rely solely on color coding of cylinders for identifying the contents. Tags and descriptive labels *must* be attached for verification; otherwise, do *not* use the cylinder. Return it to the vendor as "unidentified."
- *Always* keep cylinders chained or in a cylinder stand, whether being used or stored (Figs. 7-8, 7-9, and 7-10).
- *Never* interchange controls and fittings (designed for safety and to prevent mismatching of chemicals).
- Never completely empty a compressed-gas cylinder because of the hazard of foreign material's being sucked back into the tank.

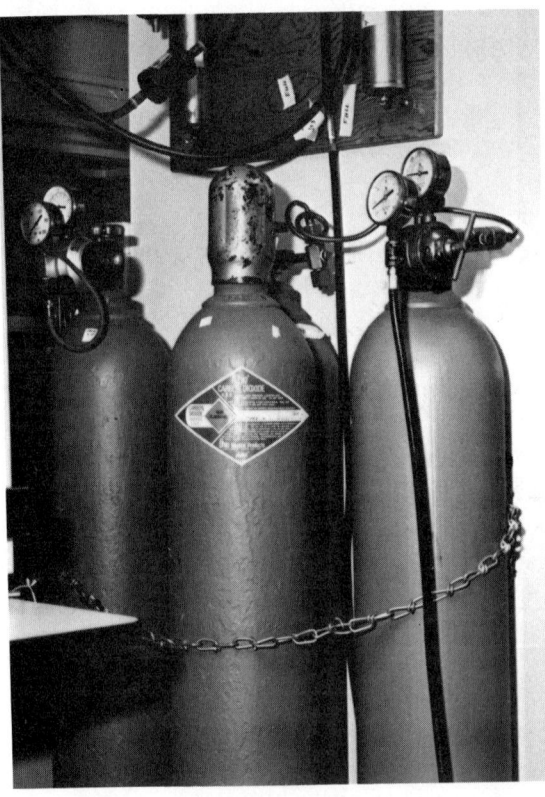

Fig. 7-8. Compressed-gas safety is very important in the laboratory. For safety, each cylinder should be chained by itself, not in groups.

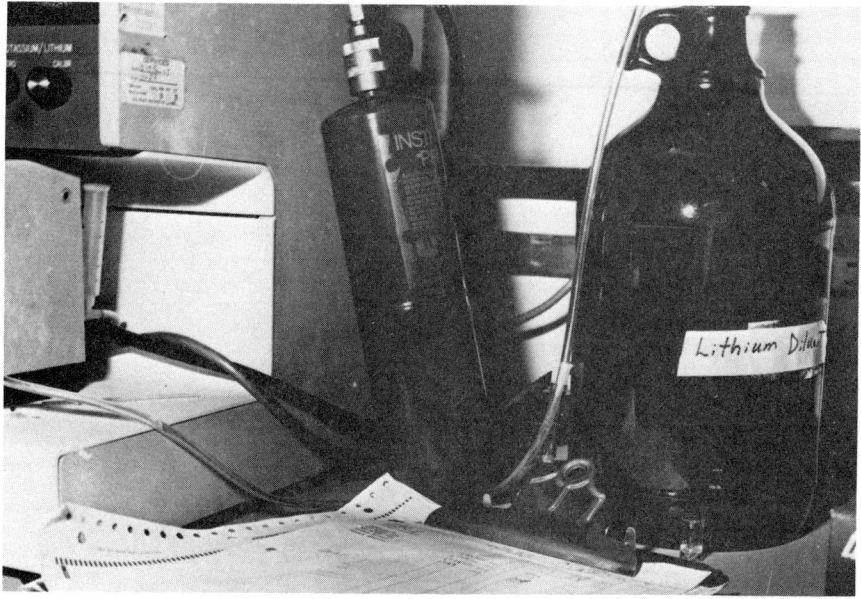

Fig. 7-9. Even a small compressed-gas cylinder of propane lying unattached against the machine where it is used represents a safety violation and a potential bomb.

- Never tamper with cylinder safety devices.
- Use the smallest cylinder size possible (Table 7-3).
- Work with all compressed gases in well-ventilated areas.
- Know the physical and physiologic properties of all compressed gases used. These include flammability, corrosiveness, toxicity, and anesthetic and irritating qualities.
- Check compressed gases for leaks before use.

Cylinder Handling

- Remember that cylinders shall be used only by trained personnel.
- Check cylinders before use by the identity tag to confirm contents.
- Always use a suitable pressure-regulating device. Close the container valve before this regulator is removed.
- Open container valves slowly and pointed them away from all

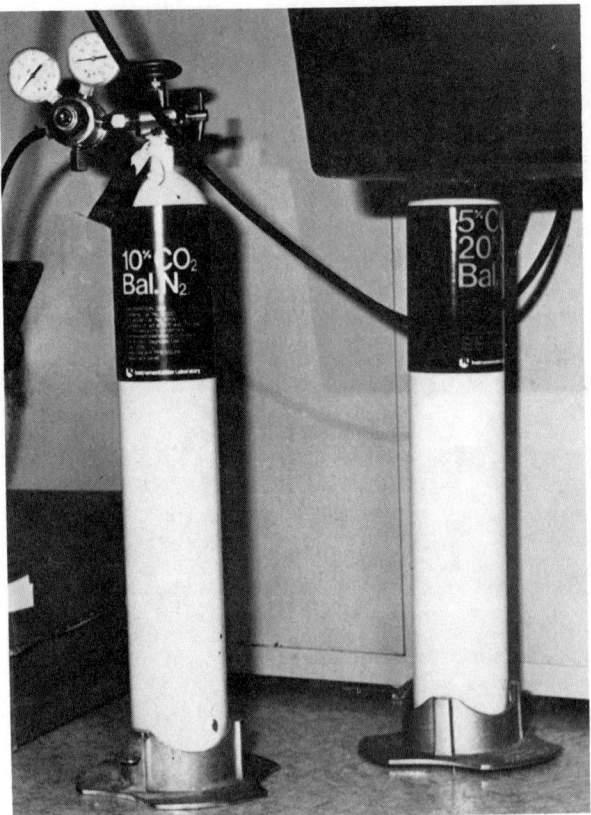

Fig. 7-10. These compressed-gas cylinders are properly stored, singly, in acceptable stands.

personnel. It is best to wear safety glasses when operating the valve.

- Never apply excess force to open a "stuck" cylinder valve.
- Test for leaks only with soap solutions.

Cylinder Storage

Ideally, cylinders should be stored in detached, well-ventilated or open-sided, fire-resistant buildings away from sources of heat, moisture, and electricity. They should be grouped by type and chained upright or horizontally. Full cylinders should be segregated from empty ones.

- Do not store containers where they may be hit by heavy objects (*e.g.,* elevators, gangways).
- Keep storage areas well equipped with fire extinguishers.
- Do *not* store standby cylinders or empty cylinders in the laboratory.

Cylinder Transportation

Cylinder valves, to which the pressure regulators are attached, are protected by valve-protector caps, which should be left in place at all times unless the cylinder is in use. The cylinder valve is thus protected from being sheared and becoming a torpedo.

Only a suitable handtruck with safety chains should be used to transport cylinders.

General Rules for Using Compressed Gases

- Do not extinguish a flame involving a combustible gas until the source of gas has been shut off.
- When they are not in use, keep cylinder and bench valves tightly closed.
- Remove regulators from empty cylinders quickly, replace the protective cap, and mark the cylinder "MT."
- Remember that oil or grease on the high-pressure side of an oxygen cylinder can cause an explosion.
- At its place of use, keep a cylinder firmly secured or placed in a cylinder stand.
- Never drop cylinders or allow them to strike each other with force.
- Remember that no part of a cylinder should be subjected to temperatures above 125°F or below −20°F or come into direct contact with a flame. Large cylinders are equipped with fusible metal safety plugs which may release if the cylinder is heated above a certain temperature. Most small cylinders do not have this protection.

(Text continues on p. 212)

Table 7-3. Respiratory Hazards of Typical Gases and Recommended Cylinder Sizes*

GAS	RESPIRATORY HAZARD†	MATHESON		AIR PRODUCTS	
		LARGEST CYLINDER	CONTENT	LARGEST CYLINDER	CONTENT
Ammonia	M	3	5 lb	D	3.4 lb
Argon	L	1A	247 cu ft	A	307 cu ft
Boron trichloride	H	LB‡	1 lb	LB	0.6 lb
Boron tri-fluoride	H	4	2 lb	LB	0.5 lb
Butadiene	L	LB	6 oz	LB	6 oz
Butane	L	LB	6 oz	LB	6 oz
1-Butene	L	LB	6 oz	LB	6 oz
2-Butene	L	LB	6 oz	LB	6 oz
Carbon dioxide	L	1A	60 lb	B	524 cu ft
Carbon monoxide	H	4	0.4 lb	D	0.7 lb
Carbonyl sulfide	H	LB	0.5 lb	LB	0.7 lb
Chlorine	H	LB	1 lb	LB	1 lb
Chlorine tri-fluoride	H	LB	1 lb	LB	1.9 lb
Dimethy-lamine	H	LB	6 oz	LB	6 oz
Dimethyl ether	L	LB	6 oz	LB	6 oz
Ethane	L	LB	4 oz	LB	5 oz
Ethylamine	H	LB	10 oz	LB	8 oz
Ethylene oxide	H	LB	8 oz	LB	8 oz
Fluorine	H	4	8 oz	D	5 oz
Helium	L	—	—	A	267 cu ft
Hydrogen	L	4	9 cu ft	D	12.8 cu ft
Hydrogen bromide	H	LB	1 lb	LB	1.2 lb
Hydrogen chloride	H	4	2 lb	D	3.7 lb
Hydrogen sulfide	H	LB	8 oz	LB	8 oz
Isobutylene	L	LB	6 oz	LB	6 oz
Methane	L	LB	6 oz	LB	—
Methylacet-ylene	L	LB	6 oz	LB	6 oz
Methyl-amine	H	LB	6 oz	LB	6 oz
Methyl bromide	H	4	7.5 lb	D	11.2 lb
Methyl chloride	H	4	3 lb	D	5.2 lb

(continued)

Table 7-3. Respiratory Hazards (continued)

GAS	RESPIRATORY HAZARD†	MATHESON		AIR PRODUCTS	
		LARGEST CYLINDER	CONTENT	LARGEST CYLINDER	CONTENT
Methyl mer-captan	M	LB	8 oz	LB	9.6 oz
Methyl vinyl ether	§	4	2.5 lb	D	4.2 lb
Nitric oxide	H	3	6 oz	D	5 oz
Nitrogen	L	1A	227 cu ft	A	280 cu ft
Nitrogen dioxide	H	LB	12 oz	LB	12 oz
Nitrous oxide	L	3	6 lb	D	0.5 lb
Oxygen	L	1A	244 cu ft	A	305 cu ft
Phosphorus penta-fluoride	H	LB	8 oz	LB	8 oz
Phosgene	H	LB	12 oz	LB	1 lb
Propane	L	LB	5 oz	LB	6 oz
P-10 (90/10 Argon–methane mixture)	L	1A	240 cu ft	—	6 oz
Sulfur dioxide	M	4	5 lb	D	7.8 lb
Sulfur hexa-fluoride	L	3	10 lb	D	6.8 lb
Trimethyl-amine	H	LB	6 oz	LB	6 oz
Vinyl bromide	M	4	5 lb	Not available	
Vinyl chloride	//	4	2.5 lb	D	4.2 lb

*Recommended largest cylinder sizes are those recommended by the supplier. Sizes are designated by Matheson in numbers and by Air Products in letters. These designations have no relation to one another or to any standard. Each size has a specific volume, diameter, and weight. Variations in content weights are due to different densities of gases.

†LOW (L): Little hazard is incurred by inhalation of airborne vapor, fumes, or dust produced during normal operations in open areas.

MODERATE (M): Inhalation of vapor, fumes, or dust may be hazardous. Prolonged or repeated exposures to low concentrations or short exposures to high concentrations are dangerous.

HIGH (H): Inhalation of vapors or fumes for even short exposure is dangerous. Approved gas masks or air-supplied respirators must be worn, or the reaction must be carried out in a hood that will eliminate all exposure.

‡Lecture bottle (LB)

§Insufficient data available to establish rating

//Carcinogen as defined by OSHA; use only under carefully controlled conditions.

(Adapted from Safety in Academic Chemistry Laboratories. American Chemical Society, 1979; used with permission)

- Use cylinders in rotation as received from the supplier.
- If a cylinder leaks and the leak cannot be remedied by the tightening of a valve, close the valve and attach a warning tag. Remove the cylinder to storage for the supplier to pick up unless it presents an immediate danger.
- On empty containers, keep valves closed and valve-protector caps in place.

8

Accidents, Emergencies, Protective Devices, and First Aid

This chapter addresses the topic of occupational accidents and their prevention and treatment. Planning for their occurrence is one of the best preventive measures and is discussed under emergency planning. The clinical laboratory is a rather unique operating facility with potentially hazardous working conditions that necessitate using special protective safety equipment and clothing. These are briefly described in this section, which includes a comprehensive listing of all relevant safety equipment and clothing currently available. This list is included to provide a resource for the newest innovations in laboratory safety devices.

For those times when an accident does take place, the final section in this chapter provides an introduction to first aid that the medical technologist might be required to use in an emergency.

ACCIDENTS AND ACCIDENT PREVENTION

A laboratory accident is any unplanned or unwanted event that results in personal injury or property damage or both and involves the release of excessive amounts of energy or hazardous materials. Accord-

213

ing to statistics kept by the Department of Labor and the National Safety Council, accidents are the leading cause of death in the United States among younger workers. For each disabling accident, there are hundreds of nondisabling accidents that do not require reporting on the Occupational Safety and Health Administration (OSHA) injury/illness forms (see Chap. 1).

By definition, minor personal injuries require only simple first aid or no treatment at all; serious injuries are those resulting in a fatality or in permanent total, permanent partial, or temporary total disability.

Accidents are usually complex, often resulting from many causes. When a detailed accident analysis takes place, one or more of the causes identified should be eliminated, preventing a recurrence. To investigate an accident properly, the following must be determined: the accident type, the energy source, the unsafe act or condition, the nature of the injury, and the affected body parts. Recommendations from these investigations can provide long- and short-range preventive measures.

The unsafe acts or conditions associated with an accident are frequently traceable to poor management policies and decisions or to personal or environmental factors. Fortunately, most laboratory managers realize that safety is both a legal and an integral part of the total laboratory operation. Most managers do take the time and the concern necessary to prepare a written safety policy; many also attempt to instill safety awareness in all their employees as a routine operating procedure. The selection, training, and placement of each employee and the purchase, inspection, and maintenance of each piece of equipment and all required supplies are considered to be as important to a successful accident-prevention program as are the maintenance of a safe and healthful environment and establishment of adequate operating and emergency procedures (see Methods for Control of Chemical, Physical, and Biological Hazards in Human Environments).

Management safety policies and decisions include management's intentions relative to safety; production and safety goals; staffing procedures; use of records; assignment of responsibility, authority and accountability; employee selection, training, placement, direction, and supervision; communication; inspections; equipment; supplies; facilities design, purchase, and maintenance; standard and emergency job procedures; and housekeeping.

Personal factors include motivation; ability; knowledge; training;

safety awareness; assignments; performance; physical and mental state; reaction time; and personal care.

Environmental factors include temperature; pressure; humidity; dust; gases; vapors; air currents; noise; illumination; electricity; radiation; ignition sources; and hazardous supports and surface objects.

In summary, accident prevention includes the establishment of safety policies, safety training, and safety-procedures review, as well as determination and correction of the direct and indirect causes of accidents. Direct causes are determined through an analysis of hazards, job safety, and incidents that occur; subsequent exposures are then reduced or further protection is provided. Indirect causes may be determined and eliminated by keeping records, making surveys, training employees, designing safer facilities, and removing unsafe conditions.

METHODS FOR CONTROL OF CHEMICAL, PHYSICAL AND BIOLOGICAL HAZARDS IN HUMAN ENVIRONMENTS

1. Elimination—removal of material or source of hazard
2. Substitution—replacement of hazard with less toxic substitute
3. Isolation—reduction of exposure by access control, barriers, containment, shielding
4. Enclosure—use of partial barrier with directed air motion
5. Ventilation—general dilution, local exhaust, make-up, and distribution of air
6. Process change—elimination or reduction of hazard or agent generation or release
7. Product change—elimination of agent, designing for safety and health
8. Housekeeping—containment, control, reduction of fugitive release
9. Dust suppression—wet methods, cleanup, vacuuming, cover re-
10. Maintenance—assurance of continued effectiveness of process, operation control
11. Sanitation—personal hygiene, washing, clean clothing, and facilities, disinfection
12. Operational practices—safety and health review and analysis
13. Education—starts with public education, knowledge of the hazard, use of engineers and designers
14. Labeling and warning systems—knowledge of where hazards are and how to avoid or reduce them

15. Personal protective devices—goggles, masks
16. Environmental monitoring—sampling and analysis for environmental action decision
17. Waste-disposal practices—disposal of hazardous wastes; disinfection; incineration
18. Administrative control—reduction of time of exposure to reduce dose
19. Medical-control program—baseline screening, biological monitoring
20. Hazard-management program—planning; organization; implementation; control

Adapted from Charles E. Billings, Ph.D., "Principles of Occupational Hygiene" (unpublished), presented here with the permission of the author at Johns Hopkins University)

Emergency Planning

An emergency occurs when safety controls fail and unforeseen circumstances occur. Every laboratory, therefore, must have a comprehensive, widely distributed, and approved emergency plan. A thorough knowledge of laboratory hazards and safety procedures is the first step in preparing personnel for emergency conditions that may arise. In addition, adequate hands-on training in using safety and fire-prevention equipment is an important factor in emergency preparedness. A typical emergency plan should have the following components:

- Ongoing programs of emergency and safety training and review for all personnel. These establish the confidence and familiarity necessary to deal with an emergency.
- Continuous evaluation and review of hazards are necessary because changes in laboratory procedures so often occur.
- Availability of proper equipment and tools for most emergencies that may arise (*e.g.,* fire, spills)
- Safety audits conducted routinely to prevent emergencies from arising and to increase safety awareness
- Familiarity of all personnel with the emergency plans
- Frequent reevaluation and updating of the emergency plans
- An evacuation plan that includes evacuation routes and shelter

areas and startup procedures for laboratory equipment, electricity, gases, and so on.

- Frequent emergency drills involving all aspects of the emergency procedures; simulated emergencies should be tested at least annually.
- Availability and proper location of alarms; periodic fire drills
- Mandatory accident, emergency, and injury reporting are required and must be permanently retained.
- Names and phone numbers of responsible personnel for each laboratory
- Emergency measures designed to emphasize prevention, containment, and cleanup procedures.
- Specialty training of certain persons in specific emergency procedures and responsibilities that they will be required to perform in an emergency. Individually designated emergency tasks include contacting responsible laboratory personnel and police, fire fighters, and medical personnel; providing necessary first aid; applying fire-fighting materials; evacuating if necessary; distributing protective equipment; and providing information to police, fire-fighters, and medical personnel.

The first actions taken in an emergency must be to alert others, to limit the spread of the danger, and to reduce or confine the hazard. In some instances, fighting the fire or remedying the situation may, of necessity, be left to professionals such as the bomb squad or fire department. In such cases, laboratory personnel can provide relevant information but should vacate the laboratory to allow the fire or other rescue personnel to perform their job and restore emergency conditions to normal.

SAFETY EQUIPMENT AND PROTECTIVE CLOTHING

It is essential that proper protective clothing be worn in the laboratory and that safety equipment be available and used when required, even when employees resist the requirement. This section covers both safety equipment and protective clothing, beginning with safety equipment (see Safety Equipment Indexed by Function and Safety Equipment Listed Alphabetically).

(Text continues on p. 224)

SAFETY EQUIPMENT INDEXED BY FUNCTION

Storage
- Cabinets
  - Acid
  - Flammables
  - Custom
  - Drum storage
  - Security
- Safety cans
- Refrigerators
- Trays
- Bench liners
- Shelf guards
- Safety racks

Safe Handling
- Carboys
- Teflon laboratory ware
- Bottle carriers
- Pipetting aids
- Safety-coated bottles
- Pumps
- Tongs
- Gas-cylinder supplies
- Laboratory carts
- Handtrucks
- Carbon caddies
- Ladders
- Vacuum cleaners
- Explosionproof equipment
- Burners
- Polynet
- Cleaners
- Bags
- Glass-disposal supplies

Personal Protection
- Respirators
  - Emergency air masks
  - Air lines
  - Escape masks
  - Gas masks
  - Chemical cartridges

Dust
Oxygen masks
Disinfection kits
Gloves
- Viton
- Neoprene
- Nitrile
- Latex
- PVA coated
- Disposal
- Glove box
- Cryo-
- Zetex
- Cal OSHA

Ear-protection equipment
- Earplugs
- Ear protectors
- Sound-level meters
- Safety caps

Eye-protection equipment
- Chemical-splash goggles
- Ultraviolet-light goggles
- Gasproof
- Visorgogs
- Protective glasses
- Sanitizers
- Lens cleaners
- Accessories
- Face shields
- Laboratory shields

Clothing
- Laboratory coats
- Aprons
- Coveralls
- Tyvek
- Boots
- Chemical-splash suits

Spill Control
- Wipers
- Absorbent paper

Mercury-control station
Mercury-vapor monitors
Mats
Hg/Vap Adsorb
Chemical neutralizers
Absorbents
Spill squeegees
Waste containers
Spill Control pillows
Universal spill kits
Spil-Karts
Spill-cleanup kits
Hazard Control
  Monitors
    Toxic gas
    Organic vapor
    Mercury vapor
    Formaldehyde
    Ethylene oxide
    Hydrogen sulfide
    Peroxide (test strips)
    *p*H paper
    Flash-point tester
    Oxygen deficiency
    Combustible gas
    Leak
    Air velocity-UV
    Electric hazard
  First Aid
    Eye washes
    Emergency showers
    Fire extinguishers
    Fire blankets
    Security
Biohazard Safety
  Biohazard bags
  Sterility indicators
  Autoclave deodorants
  Syringe-destruction equipment
  Ovens
  Disinfectants
  Biological blender top

Bacti-Cinerator II
Loops and needles
Bacteria killers
Radiation Safety
  Survey meters
  Dosimeters
  Dosimeter supplies
  Decontaminants
  Clothing, gloves
  Containers
  Shields
  Lead foil
  Liquid-solidification equipment
High/Low Temperature
  Ceramfab
    Hot pads
    Wire gauze
    Bulk fiber
    Boards
    Paper
    Cloth
  Thermometers
  Cold baths
  Refrigerant bricks
  Dewar flasks
  Dry-ice makers
Ventilation Systems
  Fume hoods
    Conventional
    Auxiliary air
    Portable
    Radioisotope
    Perchloric acid
  Biological safety cabinets
  Radioiodine traps
  Smoke generators
  Fume scrubbers
  Face velocity alarms
  Hood coatings
  Static hoods
  Fume guards

(continued)

Signs, Labels, Tapes
  Custom service
  Administration
  Chemical hazard
  Radiation hazard
  Biohazard
  Benzene
  NFPA
  Rite on chemical inventory
  Hazardous waste
  Hazard labels
  Instruction labels
  DOT labels
  Material safety data sheets
  Charts
Safety Books
  Toxic-hazardous chemicals
  Toxicology
  Safe handling
  Laboratory safety
  First aid
  Management

Adapted from Lab Safety Supply Company: Product Catalog. Janesville, WI

SAFETY EQUIPMENT LISTED ALPHABETICALLY

Absorbent paper
Absorbents
  Activated carbon
  Permasorb
  Safe N' Dri
  Vermiculite
Acid cabinets
  Epoxy steel
  Stainless steel
Acid neutralizers
Aprons
  Disposable
  Heavy duty
  Lead
  Low cost
  Plastic
  Polybutylene
  Rubber
  Tyvek
  Zetex
Autoclavable supplies
  Biohazard bags
  Carboys
  Grab bags
  Instrument/pipette pans
  Waste containers
Bacti-Cinerator II
Bag

  Holder
  Ties
Bags
  Air sampling
  Autoclavable
  Biohazard
  Hazardous waste
  Laundry, soluble
  Polycolored
  Polyethylene
  Poly liners
  Radioactive waste
  Whirl pak
Beakers, Teflon
Biohazard safety
Biological safety cabinets
Blankets
  Emergency
  Fire
  Zetex
Blenders
  Explosion proof
  Standard
Bottles
  Acid containers
  Mercury
  Plastic-coated
  Reagent

Teflon
Wash
Bulbs, pipette
Burn treatment
Burner
  Flame indicator
  Lighter
  Portable
  Safety
Cabinets
  Acid
  Biological safety
  Corrosive
  Custom
  Drum storage
  First aid
  Flammable storage
  Security
Cans, safety
  Bench
  Disposal
  Dispensing
  Drip
  Faucet safety
  Hazardous chemicals
  Lab
  Oily waste
  Plunger
  Round
  Stainless steel
  Step-on
  Tilt safety
Caps, safety
Carboy
  Autoclavable
  Safety lowboy
Carboy caddy
Carrier, radioisotope
Caustic neutralizer
Charts, safety
Chem Kleenups
Chemical neutralizers

Cleaners
  Disinfectant
  Glassware
  Hand
Clean room supplies
  Clothing
  Gloves
  Mats
  Vacuum cleaner
Cloth
  Antifog
  Ceramfab
  Flexweave
  Nomex
  Zetex
Clothing, protective
Containers, radioactive
Decontamination kit
Destruclip
Dewar flasks
Disinfectants
Dispensing cans
Dispensing jugs
Dispensers
  Drum
  Tape
Disposable wipes
Dosimeters
  Ethylene oxide
  Formaldehyde
  Hydrogen sulfide
  Mercury vapor
  Organic vapor
  Personnel protection
  Radiation
Electric pipetter
Electric receptable tester
Emergency blanket
Emergency lantern
Emergency light
Explosionproof equipment
Eye/face/body wash

(continued)

Eye-protection stations
Eye-wash stations
Face shields
Face velocity monitor
Faucet safety cans
Fill vents
Filter flask guards
Fire blankets
Fire extinguishers
First aid
Flame arrestors
Flashlight
Flash-point tester
Floor mats
   Antifatigue
   Clean room
   Conductive
Fume guard
Fume hoods
   Auxiliary air
   Conventional
   Portable
   Perchloric acid
   Radioisotope
Fume scrubber
Gas-cylinder supplies
Gas-cylinder pallet
Gas-leak detectors
Glass crushers
Glass-disposal box
Glass-tube manipulator
Glasses
   Cases
   Clip-on
   Glassblowing
   Protective
   Ultraviolet
   Visitors
Glove box
Gloves
   Animal handling
   Anticontaminant

Cal OSHA
Clean room
Disposable
Drybox
Finger cot
Glass worker's
Leaded neoprene
Leather palm
Low temperature
Natural latex
Neoprene
Nitrile
Nylon inspector's
PVA coated
Viton
Zetex
Goggles
   Chemical splash
   Encon 160
   Gasproof
   No vent
   Ultraviolet
   Visorgogs
Hg Absorb
Hg Vac
Hg Vapor Adsorb
Hot pads, Ceramfab
Hot plate, explosionproof
Inoculation loops
Instrument pans
Isoclean
Kaydry
Kleen Eyes Eyewash
Kik Step
Kim wipes
Lab coats
   Flame retardant
   General purpose
   Lab safety
   Nomex
   Office
   Polylaminated

(continued)

Oven, syringe destruction
Oversleeves
  Plastic
  Rubberized
  Tyvek
Parafilm
Penlights
Perchloric-acid fume hood
Permasorb
Peroxide test strips
pH paper
Pipettes
  Disposable
  Safety Zipp
  Zippettes
Plastic-coated bottles
Plastic coating
Polynet
Porta-Pig
Radiation dosimeters
Radiation safety equipment
Radiation survey meters
Radioiodine traps
Radioisotope carriers
Radioisotope fume hoods
Reagent bottles
Reagent trays
Refrigerators
Respirators
  Acid gas
  Air line
  Ammonia
  Cartridge
  Dust
Respirators

Organic vapor
Paint spray
Pesticides
Radionuclide
Respirator-disinfection kits
Respirator hoods
Safety cans
Safety shears
Security cabinets
Shaker, explosionproof
Shelf guards
Shields
  Face
  Pipe flange
  Safety
  Vacuum flask
Showers, emergency
Shower tester
Signs
  Administration
  Admittance
  Biohazard
  Chemical hazard
  Chemical identification
  Custom
  Danger, do not use
  Fire emergency
  First aid
  General protection
  Glow in the dark
  Lab safety
  Luminous exit
  NFPA
  No smoking
  PCB

Safety Equipment

It is usually a legal requirement as well as a safety essential to provide adequate, well-maintained safety showers, eye-wash fountains, fire extinguishers, fume hoods, and fire alarms in all clinical laboratories (Fig. 8-1). There must be a regular program of testing, inspection (every

Pipe-identification markers
Radiation hazard
Truck placards
Smoke detectors
Smoke-detector Tester
Sound-level meters
Spil-Karts
Spill-control kits
Spill Control pillows
Spill kits/disposal drums
Spill squeegees
Splash suits
  Goretex
  Vinyl
Sporicidin
Spouts
Stands, burner
Staticide
Static hood
Static meter
Sterility indicators—autoclave
Stirrers
Stop step
Support, gas cylinder
Tags
  Cylinder status
  Disposal
  Metal
Tapes
  Barricade
  Biohazard
  Broken glass
  Colored

Custom printed
Glassware
High/low temperature
Laboratory safety
Safety hazard
Teflon labware
Teflon overlay
Temperature dots
Thermometers
  Heat probe
  Nonmercury
  Surface
Tongs, safety
Toxic-gas detector
Truck
  Gas cylinder
  Hand
Ultraviolet meter
Universal spill kits
Utensils, Teflon coated
Vacuum cleaners
  Clean room
  Lab vac
  Mercury
  Wet/dry
  Shoe-brush machine
Vacuum pump, explosionproof
Wash bottles
Waste containers
Waste jugs
Watchglasses, Teflon
Wire gauze, ceramic center

Adapted with permission from Lab Safety Company: Product Catalog. Janesville, WI

3 to 6 months), repair, and maintenance to keep these items in working order and ready for the day that they might be needed. Records must be kept to verify each inspection and must be initialed by the inspector. It is also necessary that all employees be well trained in the use of safety equipment so that lack of familiarity does not add to the problem when an unforseen emergency arises. The physical area surrounding the

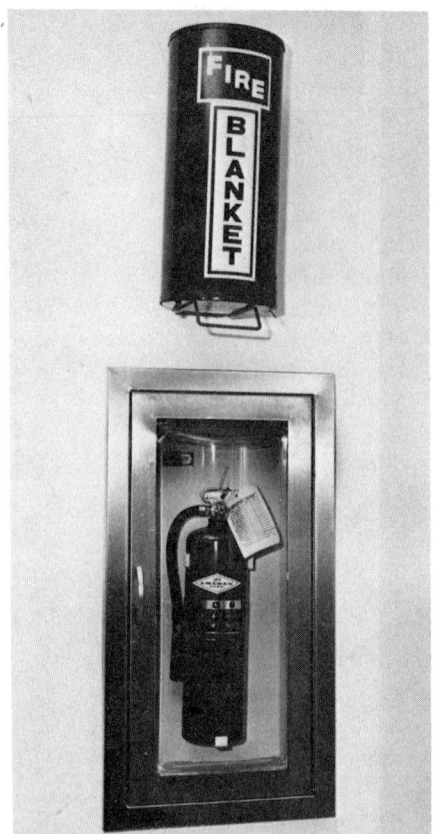

Fig. 8-1. Fire-fighting equipment must be available, accessible, and in good working order. Staff must be trained to use each piece of fire-fighting equipment.

safety equipment should be free of clutter so that access is unimpeded at all times. In addition to having the devices listed previously, a laboratory must have a well-equipped first-aid kit, a chemical-spill control kit, fire blankets, sand buckets, and, if appropriate, respirators. All safety equipment must be well marked and conveniently located. Eye washes and showers should be protected from contamination by waste materials and should deliver water of drinking purity (Figs. 8-2 and 8-3).

Fire Blankets

Current standards require that clinical laboratories have fire blankets installed. The fire blanket is a fire-fighting and personal-protection tool. If a person's clothing catches on fire, running fans the flame, so the victim should lie down and roll onto the flame to smother it. If another person is nearby, he should use the blanket to help smother the flame or treat for shock. The fire blanket is also an effective tool for escape from a burning area. It can also be used to contain and extinguish a small flammable-liquid fire or smother a small-area fire.

Self-Contained Breathing Apparatus

A self-contained breathing apparatus is suggested for all laboratory areas, and training in its use should be extended to provide 24-hour coverage. This equipment can be used in a fire situation so that per-

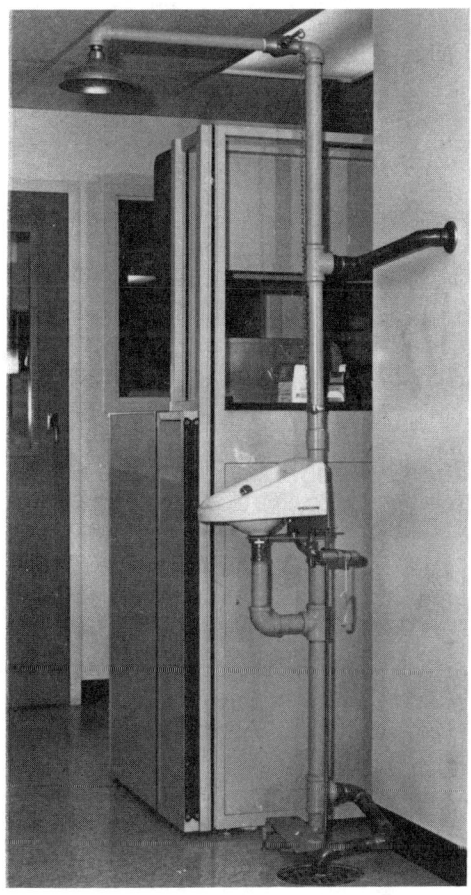

Fig. 8-2. A safety shower and eye wash combination.

sonnel wearing the apparatus can be assured that all people are out of the fire area or can don it to fight the fire. It can also be used during a chemical spill or emergency because many common chemicals produce hazardous vapors or smoke in large quantities.

Eye Wash and Shower

Emergency eye-wash and shower facilities must be available to anyone working with corrosive materials. Even mild acids and hydroxides can do serious and permanent damage if not washed off immediately.

Squeeze bottle eye washes are not recommended because of possible contamination or insufficient volume of water. They must be located within 10 seconds or 100 feet from the area where employees handle corrosives or irritants.

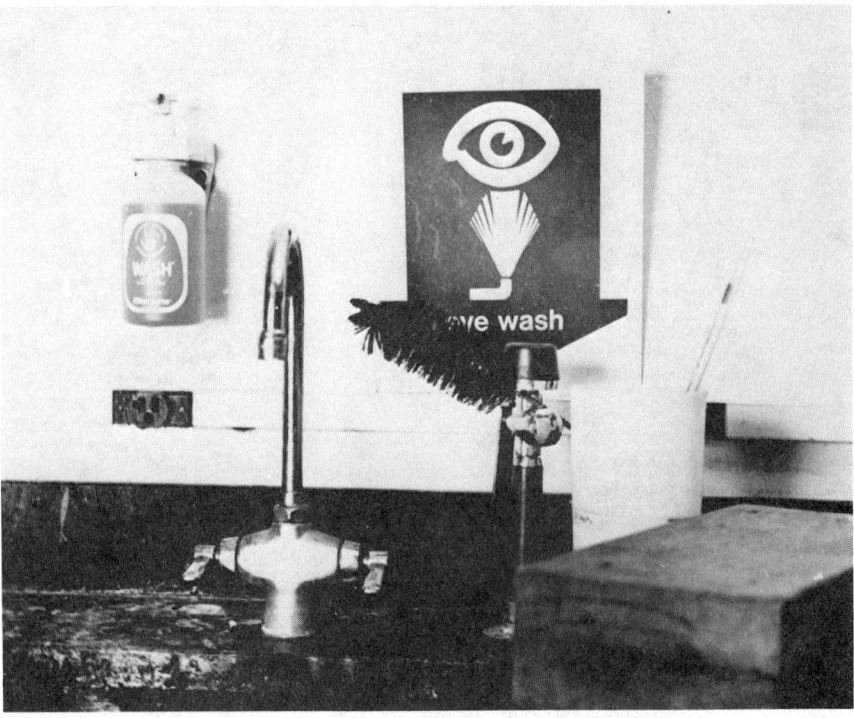

Fig. 8-3. Access to the eye wash must not be impeded. The victim cannot take time to remove objects or to grope past them while something is in the eye.

Emergency showers should be located where they can be found by someone who is disoriented. The locations of showers and eye washes should be well lit and highly visible. All employees should be instructed in the proper use of these facilities.

Protective Clothing and Apparatus

Types of protective clothing and apparatus may vary depending on the hazardous conditions of the work being performed and the rules of the laboratory. The purpose of the clothing or apparatus is to protect the body from an accidental contact with liquids, solids, or gases that may be encountered in performing laboratory procedures.

Goggles, Safety Glasses, or Face Shields

Goggles, safety glasses, and face shields are not necessary for general use but must be available when specific tasks are performed. Rigidity, strength, and the amount of protection provided are considerations in choosing the proper type of eye or face protection (Table 8-1). Contact lenses should not be worn when eye-protection equipment is used. It is the laboratory supervisor, not the technician, who will decide which procedures require eye protection. When working with ultraviolet-light sources, corrosives, chemicals, distillation apparatus, or aerosols, one can expect to be required to wear eye protection.

Gloves

Gloves must be chosen for their appropriateness to the task being performed, whether they are used to protect against burns or corrosives or broken glass. Gloves should be replaced frequently if worn; cleaned appropriately if contaminated; and inspected visually for discoloration, punctures, and tears.

Dermatitis, irritation, chemical burns, and absorption of toxic chemicals through the skin are dangerous. Hand protection can be provided only by adequate, penetration-proof gloves. Because the wearer may not always be aware of breakthrough of the liquid, the proper choice of glove characteristics as related to the chemicals to be handled is important.

[230]

Table 8-1. Comparison of Eye-Protection Devices

| TYPE | SPLASH PROTECTION | | IMPACT PROTECTION | | PROTECTION TO NECK AND FACE | COMFORT TO WEARER | ESTIMATED ACCEPTABILITY TO STUDENT | USE LIFETIME | COST |
	FRONT	SIDE	FRONT	SIDE					
Goggles	Excellent	Excellent	Excellent	Excellent	Poor	Fair	Poor	Fair	Moderate to inexpensive
Glasses (no shields)	Good	Poor	Excellent	Poor	Poor	Good to very good	Very good	Very good	Moderate
Glasses (shields)	Good	Good	Good	Fair	Poor	Good	Good	Very good	Moderate
Face shield (various sizes)	Excellent	Good to excellent	Excellent (if adequate thickness)	Good to excellent	Depends on type and length	Fair	Good for short periods	Fair	Moderate (depending on type)
Filter Lenses*									

(From Safety in Academic Chemistry Laboratories. American Chemical Society, 1979; used with permission.)

Types, Purposes, and Characteristics of Gloves

- Leather—glassware handling, broken glassware
- Cotton—general use; low abrasion resistance
- Rubber (Neoprene)—general use with fair abrasion resistance; heavy duty, virtually impervious to liquids
- Playtex—good chemical resistance, poor abrasion resistance
- Stanzoil—maximum protection from liquids; heavy duty, nonslip finish, good tear resistance
- Aluminized (NOMEX)—handling of hot materials
- Disposable vinyl or polyethylene—general use; low abrasion resistance
- Insulated (heat resistant)—handling of hot materials

Laboratory Coats

Protective clothing is advisable for most laboratory work and required by hospital policy in some situations. This clothing can include laboratory coats, aprons, and uniforms. The purpose of this apparel is to resist physical and chemical hazards without physically constraining the worker. Laboratory coats should be strong, resistant, and easily cleaned. Unfortunately, regular laboratory coats are used to protect clothing and may, if contaminated, present an added hazard such as combustibility or penetration by organic solvents.

Plastic or Rubber Aprons

Plastic or rubber aprons, or those made of other generally inert materials, provide better protection than do laboratory coats. Plastic aprons can accumulate static electricity, however, and should not be used where flammable solvents may be ignited. Disposable garments may often be preferred.

Shoes

Proper shoes should be worn in the laboratory at all times. This excludes sandals and open-toed shoes. The best shoes should provide protection against spills, slippery surfaces, and dropped objects. Laboratory policy is often lax on requirements for proper shoes, but it is an important enough concern for the employee to take the initiative and wear an appropriate nursing or laboratory shoe for his own safety.

FIRST AID

Although accidents, sudden illnesses, and other emergencies involving personnel are obviously undesirable, it is fortunate, in a sense, when they occur in the hospital laboratory because of the rapid access to physicians, nurses, and an emergency room. For this reason, one might assume that knowledge of first-aid techniques is not required for the medical technician or that a physician will always be nearby. Although this may be true, some knowledge of basic first aid is nonetheless essential for all of the laboratory staff because the seconds and minutes immediately following an accident can be used to minimize the injury or even save a life. Although a thorough course in first aid is beyond the scope of this text, some useful first-aid principles are presented. Additionally, all laboratory staff should be encouraged to take training in first aid and cardiopulmonary resuscitation (CPR).

The most common, and therefore most expected, emergency injuries in laboratories are the following:

Eye injuries from explosions, chemical burns, or particles from shattered glass or equipment
Thermal and chemical burns to skin
Cuts and puncture wounds from glass or metal with possible chemical contamination
Poisoning through the skin or by ingestion or inhalation
Chemical or electric asphyxiation

Possible adverse effects from handling chemicals include eye discomfort, breathing difficulty, dizziness, headache, nausea, vomiting, and skin irritation. In the case of any of these, work with the chemical should stop at once and supervisory personnel should be alerted.

It must be understood that first aid is only a means of providing temporary essential medical assistance until proper medical help can be obtained. The essential purposes of first aid, in order, are the following:

1. To clear the airway
2. To restore breathing and heartbeat

3. To stop bleeding
4. To prevent shock
5. To treat the wound

The initial responsibility for first aid rests with the first person at the scene. This person must begin the administration of first aid and summon help in a calm and assured manner.

General Rules for Administering First Aid

Do

- Act quickly
- Immediately alleviate respiratory arrest and severe bleeding; then focus on other injuries, wounds, fractures, burns, and so on
- Send for medical assistance
- Calm and reassure the victim
- If possible, find out from the victim and witnesses what actually occurred
- Keep the victim breathing and stop the bleeding with direct pressure
- Use artificial resuscitation to keep the victim breathing
- Know where emergency supplies are kept and where eye washes, fire blankets, and emergency showers are located
- Pull a person away from a life-threatening situation in the direction of the long axis of his body

Do Not

- Panic
- Move the victim, unless it is necessary for his safety or your own
- Leave the victim unattended
- Give the victim food, liquids, or medications until you determine the nature of the injury or illness
- Administer oxygen unless you are trained in the use of the equipment
- Attempt to straighten joints or bones
- Remove an object from the victim's eye with your finger

- Remove embedded objects from open wounds
- Break blisters on burns
- Tie a bandage or tourniquet around the victim's neck

Emergencies Requiring First-Aid Measures

Respiratory Emergencies

Respiratory emergencies are emergencies in which normal breathing is reduced or stopped and oxygen intake is insufficient to support life. Laboratory causes of respiratory emergencies can be a physical accident, circulatory failure due to shock, electric shock, and poisoning.

Restore Breathing

Signs of breathing impaired by a foreign object in the throat are the following:

- Gasping for air
- Violent fits of coughing
- Turning blue
- Inability to talk or breathe

Methods of *first-aid treatment* in such cases follow:

- Open the victim's mouth and grasp and remove the object.
- Place the head lower than the body or roll the victim onto his side and slap him on the back.
- Stand behind the victim and place your arms above the victim's navel and below his rib cage. Lean the victim forward in a hanging position. Grasp your own wrist and exert sudden strong pressure against the victim's abdomen to expel the obstruction.

When breathing is impaired from other causes, **signs** are the following:

- No detectable rise and fall of chest or abdomen
- No detectable expulsion of air from the nose or mouth

First-aid treatment in such cases follows (only one example will be given, although there are several other methods):

- Mouth-to-mouth (mouth-to-nose) resuscitation (Fig. 8-4)
- Work quickly and continue until the victim breathes normally or is pronounced dead.
- Place the victim on his back, chin up.
- Use your fingers to remove any possible obstruction, making sure that the victim's tongue is not blocking the airway.

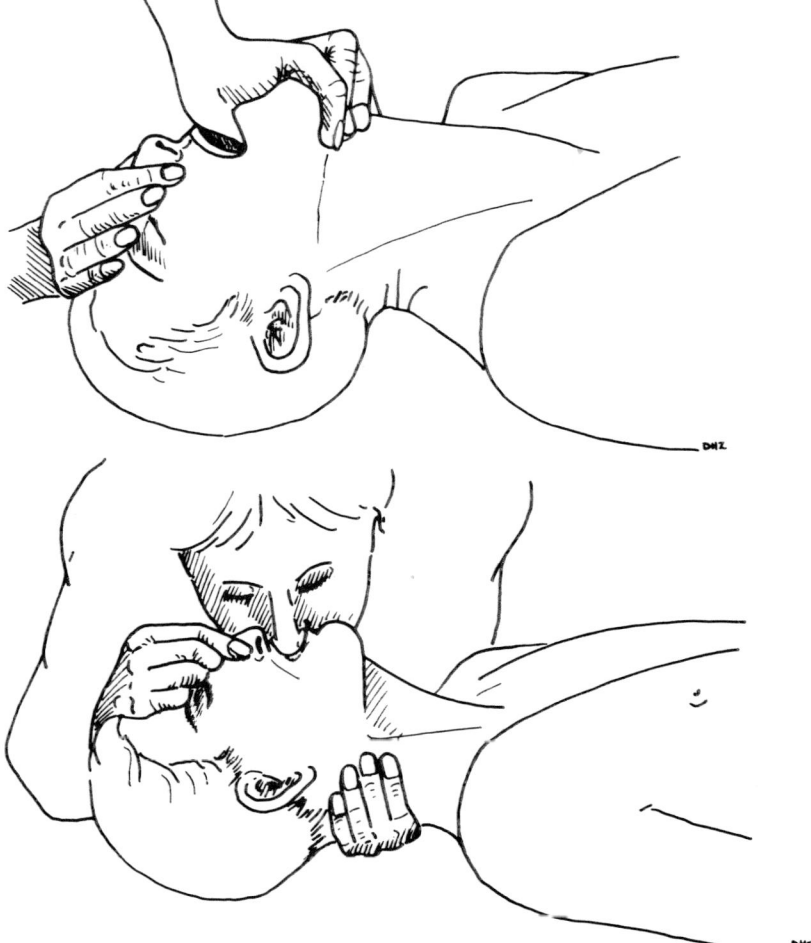

Fig. 8-4. Mouth-to-mouth (mouth-to-nose) method.

- Kneel at the victim's side, pinching the nose closed (or the mouth, in mouth-to-nose) to form an airtight seal and breathe into the mouth until the chest expands. Breathe three times. Repeat the process. If no air exchange begins, turn the victim onto his side and slap him between his shoulder blades. Again, check the mouth for an obstruction and repeat the whole breathing procedure. Do not forget to remove your mouth after each breath to allow the air to escape.

Circulatory Failure

Circulatory failure is a result of the lack of pumping action by the heart. It can occur as a consequence of other emergency conditions such as electric shock, respiratory obstruction, or heart attack.

Signs

- No breathing
- No pulse

First-Aid Treatment

- Work quickly—cardiac arrest may mean death to the victim.
- Check for responsiveness, then check airways and breathing.
- If the victim is not breathing, give four quick breaths, mouth-to-mouth.
- Check a major artery to find a pulse. If there is none, begin the following
  - Cardiac-compression procedure (Fig. 8-5)
    - Kneel at the victim's side. The pressure point for cardiac compression is two fingers' distance above the tip of the sternum. Place the heel of the hand at this point and the other hand over the first one.
    - Positioning your shoulders over the victim's sternum, rock your weight downward, depressing the sternum 1.5 inches to 2 inches, making the depressing and releasing of equal length of time.
    - Compressions should be continued at the rate of approxi-

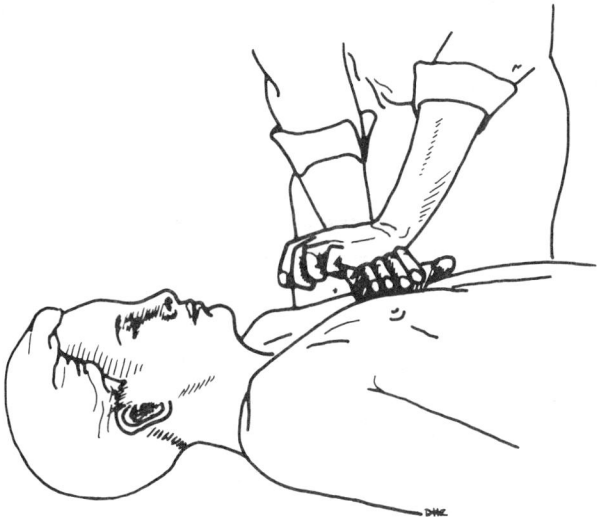

Fig. 8-5. Cardiac compressions.

mately 60 compressions per minute, with an artificial-resuscitation breath every 15th compression.

Bleeding

Bleeding results from a wound or break in the body tissue and may be internal or external. In the laboratory, bleeding usually results from mishandling of sharp objects, falling, or being struck by glass fragments.

External Bleeding

Signs of external bleeding are blood's spurting, flowing, or oozing from an artery, vein, or capillary.

First-aid treatment for external bleeding is as follows:

- Cover the wound with the cleanest cloth available (or bare hand) and apply direct pressure to the wound.
- If there is no fracture, elevate the limb as pressure is applied.
- Digital pressure may also be applied if the wound is an arterial wound and the bleeding is severe. Pressure should be applied where the main artery supplies the wound as close as possible to

the wound and between the wound and the heart. Hold the pressure point tightly for approximately 5 minutes. If there is a skull injury and direct pressure cannot be applied, use the pressure points.

- A tourniquet should be used as a last resort and should be applied near the wound, between the wound and the point at which the limb is attached to the body. Do not tie it too tightly; tie it just tightly enough to stop the bleeding. Never apply a tourniquet directly over a wound.
- Open wounds should be protected from infection by covering them with a clean fabric.

Internal Bleeding

Signs of internal bleeding are the following:

- Cold, clammy skin
- Weak, rapid pulse
- Eyes dull and pupils enlarged
- Thirst
- Nausea, vomiting
- Pain

First-aid treatment for internal bleeding is as follows:

- Treat for shock.
- Give nothing by mouth.
- Get medical help quickly.

Shock

Shock is a condition resulting from depression of vital body functions; it may be life threatening. It may result from a loss of blood volume, reduced blood flow, or insufficient oxygen supply. Traumatic shock results from an injury; anaphylactic shock results from an allergic reaction to a foreign substance.

Signs

- Shallow breathing
- Rapid, weak pulse
- Nausea, vomiting
- Shivering
- Confusion
- Drooping eyelids
- Dilated pupils
- Pale, moist, cold skin

First-Aid Treatment

- Remove cause of shock if possible.
- Establish and maintain the airway.
- Control bleeding.
- Keep the victim flat.
- Cover the victim to keep him warm.
- Give nothing by mouth.
- If appropriate, elevate the victim's feet.

Electric Shock

Electric shock results from the passage of an electric current through any part of the body.

Signs

Depending on the amount of current received, signs may include the following:

- Unconsciousness
- Visible burns where contact occurred
- Shallow breathing, as in shock
- Irregular heart rate, fibrillation
- Central nervous system damage

First-Aid Treatment

- Shut off the current or cautiously, using an insulator (*e.g.,* hand inside a glass beaker), separate the victim from the current.
- Begin artificial respiration.
- Keep the victim warm.

Poisoning

Poisoning is due to any substance that impairs health or causes death when introduced into the body or onto the skin surface. In the laboratory, poisoning is due to ingestion, inhalation, or absorption through the skin.

Signs

- Telltale odor on breath
- Burns around the mouth
- Wide variety of signs depending on the poison and the mode of ingestion or intoxication—generally a change from the normal (*e.g.,* dilated pupils, nausea, impaired breathing)

First-Aid Treatment

When poisoning is through ***ingestion*** of a toxic substance, first-aid treatment is as follows:

- Dilute or neutralize the poison.
- If the poison is ingested and is noncorrosive, dilute it with milk or water by mouth.
- Induce vomiting unless the poison is a petroleum product.
- If feasible, administer the correct antidote.
- For corrosive poisons, do not induce vomiting; give milk or water.
- If necessary, treat for shock.

When poisoning is through ***inhalation*** of a toxic substance, first-aid treatment is as follows:

- Remove the victim from the area.
- Loosen clothing.

- Clear the airways.
- Initiate artificial respiration.
- Keep the victim warm.

When poisoning is through *skin contact* with a toxic substance, first-aid treatment is as follows:

- Remove the victim's clothing and drench the victim.
- Wash contaminated skin with soap and water for a minimum of 5 minutes if tissues have not been badly destroyed.
- Administer artificial respiration if required.

Bone and Joint Injuries

Broken bones or fractures are either simple (no open wound) or compound (associated with an open wound and protruding bone). Injuries to the skeletal system and joints, ligaments, and soft tissues are common in major accidents.

Signs

- Broken bones, with no open wound
- Open fracture, deformity, swelling, discoloration
- Separation of two bones—deformity, pain, loss of function

First-Aid Treatment

- Leave the injury alone—do not attempt to straighten the limb.
- Try to immobilize the victim in a comfortable position.
- Obtain assistance.
- Stop the bleeding.

Burns

A burn is an injury resulting from contact with heat, chemicals, or radiation. The goals are to reduce pain, prevent contamination, and treat for shock.

Signs

- Red skin—first degree
- Red skin, blisters—second degree
- Skin destroyed, tissues charred and damaged—third degree

First-Aid Treatment

For first-degree burns, immerse the burn in cold water and apply ice.

For second-degree burns, cut away the clothing, cover the burn with cold, moist dressings, and treat for shock. Do not disturb blisters.

For third-degree burns, treat the victim as follows:

- Cut away loose clothing that is *not* attached to the wound.
- Cover the wound with sterile, cold, moist dressings, taking care to keep burned areas from contact with each other.
- Do not apply ointments, ice, or salves on open blisters.
- For chemical burns, remove clothing and flood the area for at least 15 to 20 minutes.

Eye Injuries

Eye injuries are a common laboratory emergency. All personnel should know where eye washes are located. Contact lenses should not be allowed when there is a chemical-splash hazard. Protective eyeglasses should be used in the laboratory.

Foreign Body or Chemical in Eye

Signs of injury due to a foreign object or chemical in the eye include the following:

- Redness
- Burning
- Tearing
- Blinking

First-aid treatment for such injuries is as follows:

- Do not rub the eye.
- Remove contact lenses at once because they may retain the chemical or object and prevent adequate flushing.
- Have the victim flush eyes well for at least 15 minutes, with assistance, holding eyelids open and apart.
- If possible, remove the foreign object with sterile gauze. If you are unable to do so, cover the eye (but not with cotton) and obtain medical assistance.

Impaled Object in Eye

Signs of an impaled object in the eye include the following:

- Object may be visible protruding from eye
- Blinking
- Tearing
- Pain
- Bleeding

First-aid treatment for such injuries is as follows:

- Do not attempt to remove the object.
- Cover the injured eye lightly with a gauze bandage.
- Place covering over both eyes (because both eyes move synchronously) to stop movement.
- Calm the victim and obtain medical assistance.

9
Laboratory-Waste Handling and Disposal

Laboratory-waste generation and disposal represent all of the hazards, chemical, biological, and radiologic, that may be present in the laboratory; in addition, they represent a potential economic and regulatory burden. Hospital laboratories are subject to increasingly complex codes and regulations with regard to waste disposal, and prospects are that these regulations will increase further in number and complexity in the future. This chapter discusses these regulations and provides some guidelines for proper waste handling and disposal. Once waste leaves the laboratory for an incinerator, landfill, or hazardous-waste site, the laboratory is *not* relieved of the responsibility for safe and legal handling. The laboratory or hospital management must assure that the commercial disposal firm is properly licensed and appropriate for the job requested. The generator of the waste bears the legal responsibility for its final disposal.

The major issue in waste handling, other than the legal aspects, is the health-and-safety issue. Careless actions endanger maintenance and housekeeping crews as well as unsuspecting workers. Paying proper attention to waste handling safeguards the entire hospital staff, patients, visitors, and the community at large.

PLANNING

Safe and environmentally sound laboratory-waste disposal begins with a well thought out, written plan that is the result of a comprehensive analysis of what comes into the laboratory (supplies, specimens, equipment) and what must eventually be discarded as waste (very broadly everything that is not kept, used up, returned, or reused). Special handling for hazardous, chemical, infectious, and radioactive wastes must all be detailed in the plan. Adequate separation and disposal of "safe" waste needs to be considered and addressed. Implementing the waste disposal plan necessitates a set of strictly enforced, detailed, and unambiguous rules and policies by which the staff must operate on a day-to-day basis.

An adequate amount of equipment be provided to carry out these plans. *All* waste that is generated must be treated or disposed of as soon as possible after it is generated (Fig. 9-1). Waste must not be allowed to accumulate. Adequate planning also involves substituting nonhazardous for hazardous materials whenever possible, using procedures calling for minimum quantities of hazardous materials, and storing only small amounts of hazardous materials beyond those immediately needed.

REGULATORY ASPECTS OF WASTE DISPOSAL

One major piece of federal waste legislation that may have greater impact on the clinical laboratory in the future than it does now is the Resource Conservation and Recovery Act of 1976 (RCRA). It was designed to require safe management of hazardous materials from their creation to their final disposal, or "from cradle to grave." Wastes that are not considered hazardous are treated much less stringently, although they do come under a variety of other federal and local laws.

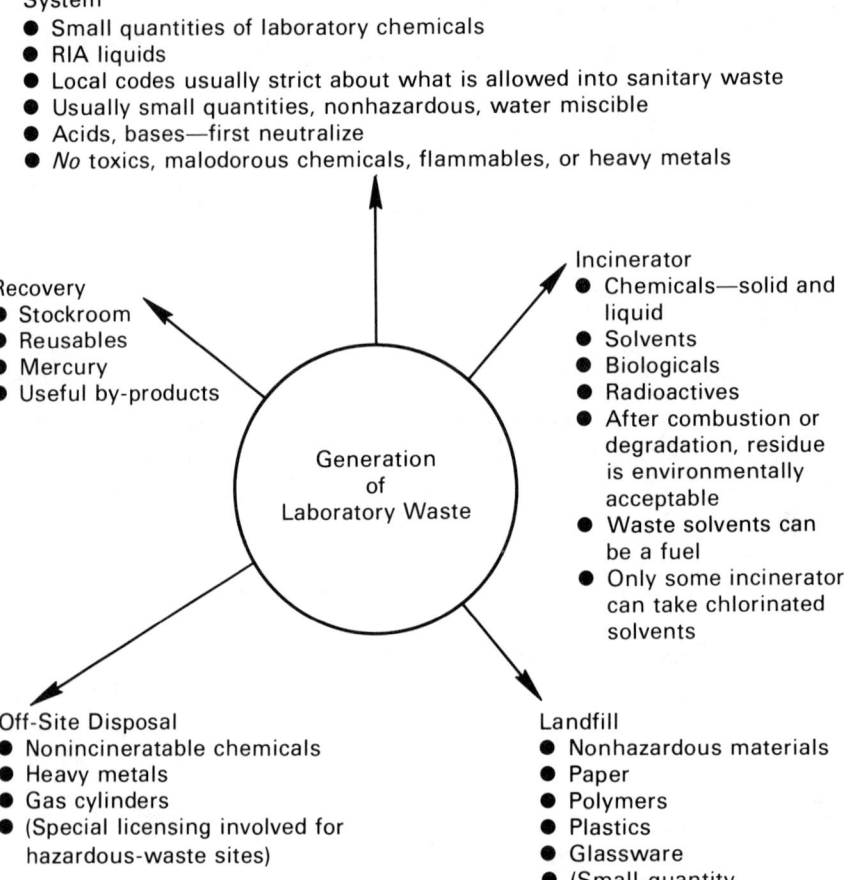

Sanitary or Sewage System
- Small quantities of laboratory chemicals
- RIA liquids
- Local codes usually strict about what is allowed into sanitary waste
- Usually small quantities, nonhazardous, water miscible
- Acids, bases—first neutralize
- *No* toxics, malodorous chemicals, flammables, or heavy metals

Recovery
- Stockroom
- Reusables
- Mercury
- Useful by-products

Generation
of
Laboratory Waste

Incinerator
- Chemicals—solid and liquid
- Solvents
- Biologicals
- Radioactives
- After combustion or degradation, residue is environmentally acceptable
- Waste solvents can be a fuel
- Only some incinerators can take chlorinated solvents

Off-Site Disposal
- Nonincineratable chemicals
- Heavy metals
- Gas cylinders
- (Special licensing involved for hazardous-waste sites)

Landfill
- Nonhazardous materials
- Paper
- Polymers
- Plastics
- Glassware
- (Small-quantity generators of hazardous waste may dispose of them in landfill if landfill operator permit allows)

Fig. 9-1. Examples of laboratory-waste management possibilities.

Clinical laboratories, because they do not generate more than 1000 kg/mo of hazardous wastes, are exempted from RCRA as small generators of hazardous waste. This may change, but at this time it does allow for laboratory waste to be disposed of through municipal sewers and landfills. RCRA does not preempt state and local regulations that are more stringent. Some states, for example, regulate hazardous-waste generators of as little as 100 kg/mo. Thirty-four states have hazardous-waste plans authorized by the Environmental Protection Agency (EPA).

For nonhazardous as well as hazardous waste, state and local regulations often provide specific disposal requirements for hospitals and laboratories. These regulations are often more restrictive than are related federal laws. For example, the Nuclear Regulatory Commission (NRC) and the EPA allow the materials used in radioimmunoassay (RIA) procedures to be discarded in sinks or in solid municipal waste. The city of Washington D.C., however, requires special disposal of the solid RIA waste.

For a waste generator to be regulated by RCRA, a determination must be made as to the hazardous nature of the waste. The waste generator must determine the following:

> Is the material solid *waste*? Remember, this is not clearcut; some materials may be reused or are usable by-products. In either case, they are not waste. Regulated waste is something destined for a landfill, *not* a sink.
>
> Is the material *hazardous*? Is it excluded by the law? Is it listed by the law? Is it a mixture of solid waste and listed waste? Does it have hazardous characteristics? Is it ignitable or corrosive ($pH < 2$ and > 12.5)? Remember that infectious waste is not yet regulated under RCRA.
>
> Is the laboratory excluded as a small operator (< 1000 kg/mo)?

Several other federal regulations and guidelines pertain to hazardous properties of waste and these must also be taken into consideration by the laboratory. For example, the EPA hazardous-waste regulations address the toxic, ignitable, corrosive, and reactive properties of wastes; NRC guidelines address radioactive properties; and EPA guidelines written under the Toxic Substances Control Act address the total management of certain chemicals.

WASTE-REMOVAL CONTRACTORS

If the amount of waste generated is *not* hazardous and is greater than 1000 kg/mo, any vendor registered to receive municipal wastes may be hired to remove the waste. Under RCRA, only those waste-disposal operators licensed by EPA and the Department of Transportation (DOT) may be hired to remove *hazardous* waste. For all waste, but most especially hazardous waste, it is essential to know the vendor—liability remains with the waste *generator* for safe and legal disposal.

METHODS OF WASTE DISPOSAL

The rest of this chapter addresses the proper handling and precautions for sharp-waste disposal, biohazardous waste disposal (infectious waste disposal), chemical-waste disposal, and radioactive-waste disposal (Fig. 9-2).

Sharp-Waste Disposal

One of the unique problems found in a health-care environment is the abundance of needles and other sharp objects ("sharps"), most of which are expected to be used once and then discarded. Sharps possess a physical-injury hazard as well as an infection hazard. Standards require that they be handled differently from ordinary trash. Objects in the category include blood-drawing equipment, hypodermic needles, syringes, Pasteur pipettes, broken glass, and scalpel blades.

The key to effective control of these wastes is to have disposal sites immediately available at the point of use (Fig. 9-3). The wastes should be packaged in such a way to eliminate the possibility of contact during subsequent handling, treatment, and disposal. After use, sharps should be placed directly into special containers. Needles should not be recapped because of the possibility of injury by self-inoculation. Contaminated needles should not be broken or clipped unless the clipping device effectively contains aerosols and needle parts, so that aerosol generation or airborne needle parts do not become an additional hazard. Containers for sharps should be impervious, rigid, and punctureproof. Suitable materials for sharps containers include glass, metal, rigid plastic, wood, and heavy cardboard. Sharps containers should be sealed, marked with the universal biohazard symbol, and autoclaved. They may then be ground up or buried in a landfill.

One management system for handling disposable sharps involves placement of used sharps directly into pans of disinfectant, followed by steam sterilization treatment and subsequent clipping of the treated needles and syringes. Although this type of treatment removes the infection hazard, the hazard of physical injury from the sharps nonetheless remains. Because of the potential for physical injury, it is not prudent to retrieve needles from a loaded pan, to handle them, or to clip them.

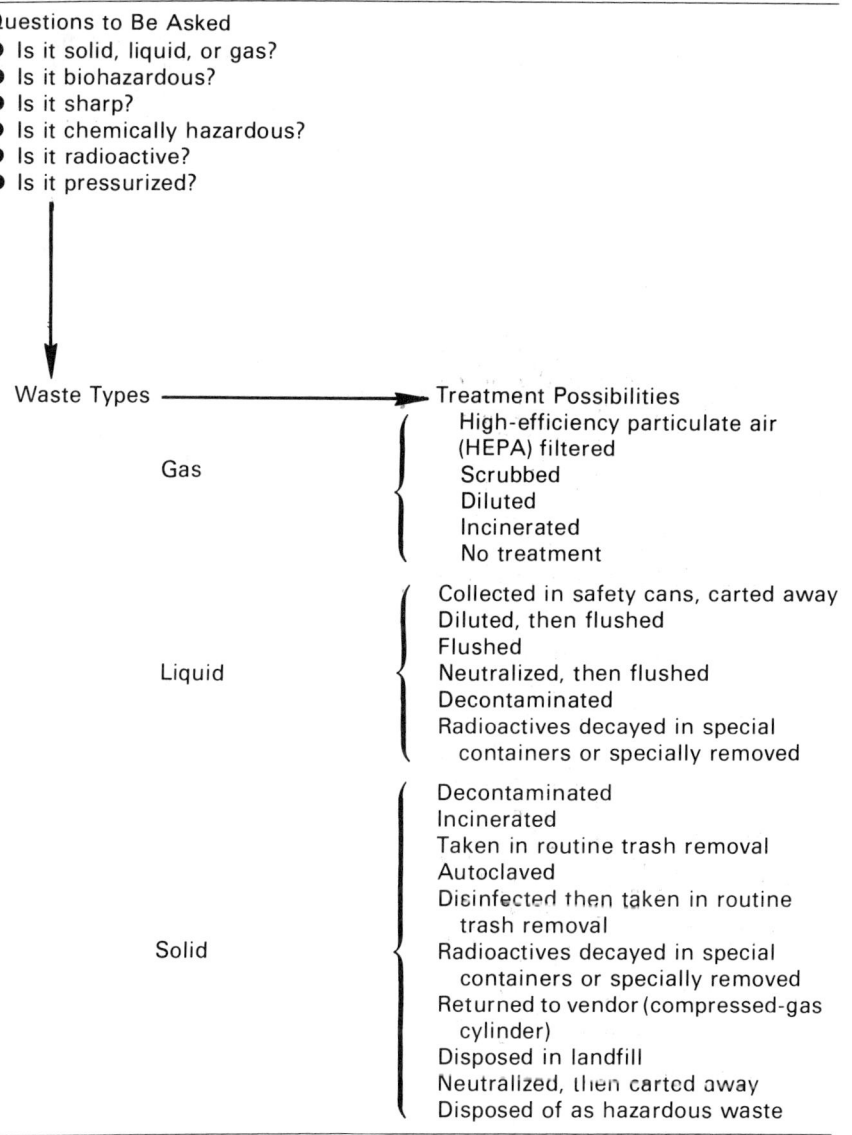

Questions to Be Asked
● Is it solid, liquid, or gas?
● Is it biohazardous?
● Is it sharp?
● Is it chemically hazardous?
● Is it radioactive?
● Is it pressurized?

Waste Types ──────────────► Treatment Possibilities

Gas

High-efficiency particulate air (HEPA) filtered
Scrubbed
Diluted
Incinerated
No treatment

Liquid

Collected in safety cans, carted away
Diluted, then flushed
Flushed
Neutralized, then flushed
Decontaminated
Radioactives decayed in special containers or specially removed

Solid

Decontaminated
Incinerated
Taken in routine trash removal
Autoclaved
Disinfected then taken in routine trash removal
Radioactives decayed in special containers or specially removed
Returned to vendor (compressed-gas cylinder)
Disposed in landfill
Neutralized, then carted away
Disposed of as hazardous waste

Fig. 9-2. An approach to waste handling.

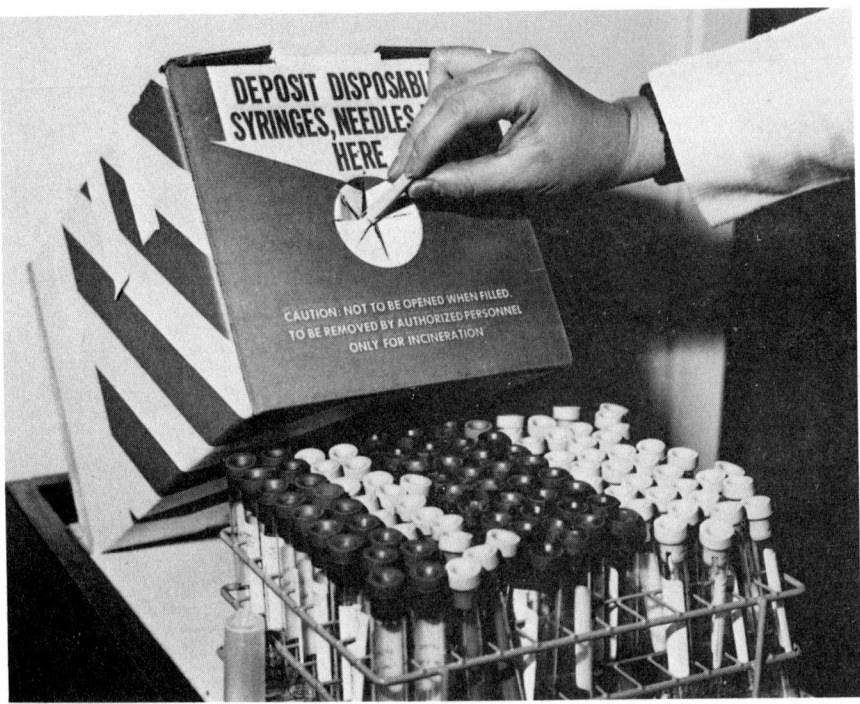

Fig. 9-3. Immediate disposal of sharps in an impervious container is the preferred method. The container will then be autoclaved.

Although waste needle and other sharps handling procedures may vary, autoclaving or incineration is mandatory to remove the infection hazard. Final disposal should provide assurance that these materials *cannot* be retrieved. Landfill is the best final disposition.

A typical injury rate from sharps is 15/mo for a 475-bed hospital with an average cost of $65 per injury. With good management practices, the hazards of disease and injury from sharps can be minimized. All waste sharps should be managed uniformly in accordance with the practices established for infectious sharps.

Biohazardous-Waste Disposal

One of the major hazards of working in the clinical laboratory is the contact with infectious material. Safe handling of infectious or biohazardous materials does *not* end until the materials are effectively decontaminated and then can be discarded with routinely disposed materials. Additional treatment is necessary, however, for such wastes as sharps, pathology specimens, and wastes with multiple hazards.

Some common contaminated laboratory wastes include the following:

Culture dishes
Pipettes
Needles and other sharps
Tissue-culture bottles and flasks
Membrane filters
Collection containers from specimens of all blood, body fluids, body
    wastes, and tissues
Microtiter plates used for hemagglutination testing, complement
    fixation testing, or antibody titer testing
Slides and plates from immunodiffusion testing
Slides and coverslips from blood specimens or tissue or colony
    picking
Disposable rubber gloves, laboratory coats, and aprons
Swabs and loops used in microbiology
Assemblies used for diagnostic purposes to speciate enteric or other
    pathogens
Centrifuge tubes

In the past, state regulations of infectious waste has been carried out by state health departments. Since the passage of RCRA, many states have passed hazardous-waste statutes that give the state authority to control infectious waste. Only some states have actually promulgated regulations controlling infectious waste. In many states, infectious waste is controlled under solid-waste laws. In addition, hospitals and nursing homes may have specific infectious-waste control requirements. The perceived dangers and proper handling of infectious waste vary greatly among the states.

Suggested Procedures for Biohazardous-Waste Handling (Fig. 9-4)

1. All laboratory specimens or materials consisting of, containing, or contaminated with blood, plasma, serum, urine, feces, or other human or animal tissues or fluids, as well as inoculated media, cultures, and other potentially infectious materials, must be either incinerated or sterilized

by autoclaving (or by use of a chemical sterilant when incineration or autoclaving is not possible).

2. When there is no reasonable evidence to indicate that clinical specimens or other materials may contain an infectious agent, disposal into a sewer without sterilization may be permitted. Materials that may be discarded directly into a sewer include uninoculated liquid mediums, tissue cultures, and nutrient fluids; and serum, plasma, or blood provided that the specimens are not believed to contain any infectious agent.

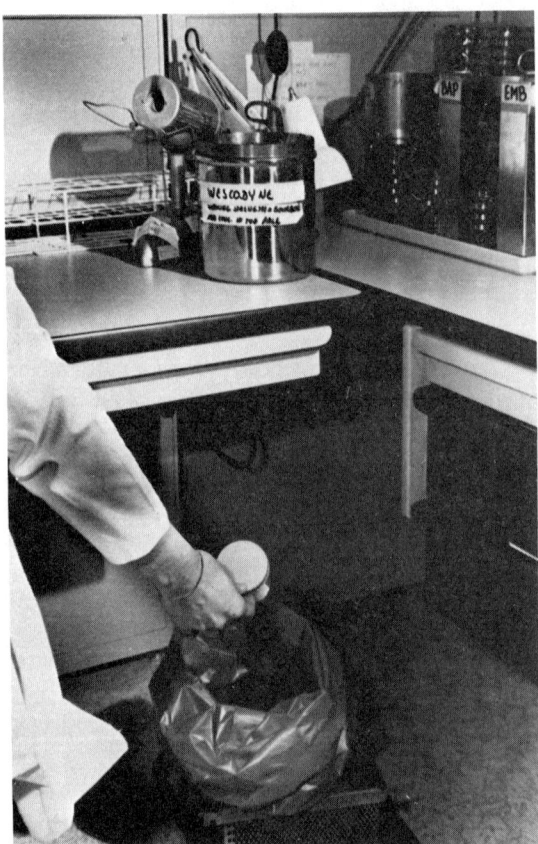

Fig 9-4. Containers of liquid disinfectant and biohazard bags should be available at each microbiology work station. Procedures should clearly delineate what type of waste goes into each.

3. All glassware, pipettes, slides, and so on, used in the examination or testing of biological materials must be autoclaved or chemically disinfected before being discarded or prepared for reuse. Single-use bottles, tubes, vials, and other biological-specimen containers should not be placed in wastebaskets that are customarily emptied by the housekeeping staff.

4. Any breakage of bags or leakage of contaminated materials should be reported to the laboratory supervisor at once for instructions on procedures for safe cleanup.

5. Detailed instructions about wastes that contain radioactive materials are available from the radiation safety officer.

6. Proper handling of sharps includes discard directly into impervious, rigid, punctureproof containers and placement of intact needles directly into collection containers with no recapping, clipping, or breaking.

7. Discard of liquid infectious waste should be in capped or tightly stoppered bottles and flasks.

8. All containers must be marked with the universal biohazard symbol (and with other labels, as necessary, to denote multiple hazards).

9. There should be no compaction of infectious waste or packages of infectious waste prior to treatment.

10. Packaging materials used should be appropriate for the type of treatment.

11. Packaging materials used should be strong enough to remain intact during whatever type of handling, storage, and transfer the packages may undergo.

12. Plastic bags used should be seamless, impervious, and tear resistant and should be red or orange in color to contain many types of infectious wastes (the principal exceptions to this disposal color are sharps and liquids).

13. Waste should be double-bagged or placed in a bag within a rigid or semirigid container in order to protect the integrity of the packaging when infectious waste is moved.

14. All infectious-waste containers should be clearly marked with the universal biohazard symbol, and plastic-bag inserts into metal waste containers should be red or orange.

Red and orange colors are used to identify biological hazards. Plastic bags of these colors are *not* to be used for noninfectious waste. Color segregation, perhaps with differently shaped metal containers, is recommended (Fig. 9-5).

15. *Reusable* items that are infectious should be placed after use directly into a separate container and disinfected immediately. They may be placed horizontally into a pan of chemical disinfectant.

16. Wastes characterized by mixed hazards should be discarded as suitable for the type of waste and type of hazard.

17. Infectious waste should be separated from general, non-

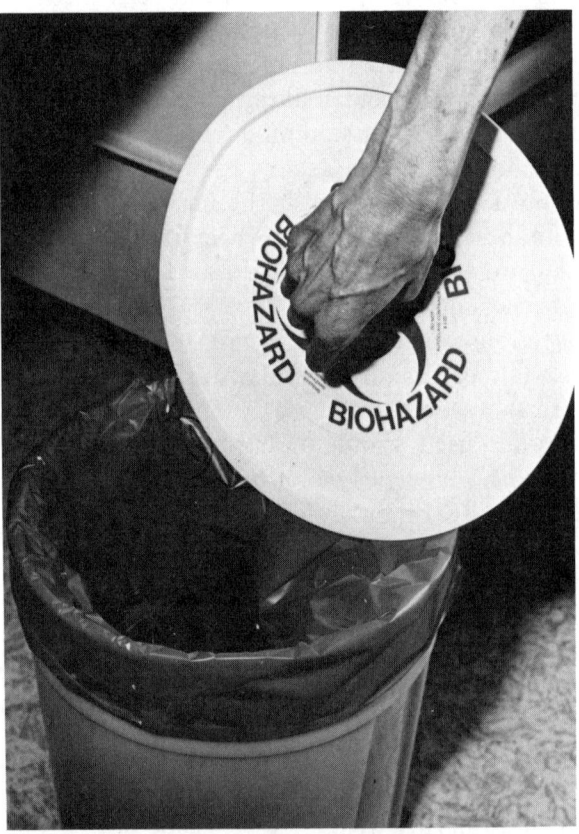

Fig. 9-5. A well-labeled biohazardous-waste container.

infectious waste at the source where the infectious material becomes a waste. Those who work with the infectious materials are most qualified to assess the hazard, and separation at this stage minimizes further handling and exposure.

Chemical-Waste Disposal

Proper disposal of chemicals is a responsibility of all laboratory workers. Arrangements for disposal may vary from laboratory to laboratory, depending on the facilities and the types of substances used, but the substances must be disposed of in ways that avoid harm to people and the environment. Also, wastes should be transferred in a form that is safe and acceptable to the people involved in disposal operations.

Very hazardous substances may be converted into less hazardous substances in the laboratory rather than being placed directly into containers. Highly reactive substances, such as metallic sodium and peroxides, should be converted into less reactive substances. Reactions may be moderated by dilution, cooling, or the slow addition of a neutralizing agent. For water-miscible materials, pouring the reaction mixture onto a bed of ice can often be a way to cool and dilute it simultaneously.

Known Neutralization Methods for Chemical Waste

Chemical waste—solid, liquid, or gas—should first be neutralized according to accepted methods to eliminate its hazardous properties. The neutralized waste, depending on its physical state, may then be disposed of by being poured into a chemical sink, exhausted slowly into an operating fume hood, or placed in a noncombustible waste can. It is the responsibility of the laboratory to make every effort to dispose of waste in this manner.

The Sewer System

Sewer systems operate in various ways, and some of them may be harmed or may present hazards when certain chemicals are added directly. Local regulations usually address what may be poured down the drain. The laboratory supervisor should know the local regulations and communicate this information to the laboratory workers. All laboratory workers should know and conform to these regulations. For sewer systems that discharge into waterways, federal regulations limit the disposal of certain toxic chemicals. The following rules regarding disposal into a sewer system should be observed:

- Only water-soluble substances should be disposed of in the laboratory sink. Solutions of flammable solvents in amounts under 1 liter must be sufficiently diluted so that they do not pose a fire hazard. Adequate dilution is *not* provided by pouring undiluted waste into a sink and then flushing. Larger quantities than 1 liter may not be disposed of through the sink.
- Strong acids and bases should be diluted to the *p*H of range 3 to 11 before they are poured in the sewer system. Acids and alkalis should not be poured into the sewer drain at a rate exceeding the equivalent of 50 ml of concentrated substance per minute.
- Highly toxic, malodorous, or lachrymatory chemicals should not be disposed of in a drain. Laboratory drains are generally interconnected; a substance that goes down one sink may well come up as a vapor in another.
- There is a hazard of contact of chemicals from two sources with one another; the sulfide poured into one drain may contact the acid poured into another, with unpleasant consequences. Some simple reactions may even cause explosions (*e.g.,* ammonia plus iodine, silver nitrate plus ethanol, or picric acid plus lead salts).
- Small amounts of some heavy-metal compounds may be disposed of in a sink, but larger amounts may pose a hazard for the sewer system or water supply. Check local regulations.

Solid Chemical Wastes

Each institution should have procedures for collecting solid chemical wastes from its laboratories and arranging for disposal. A statement as to who is in charge and the responsibilities of the laboratory workers for identification of hazards that may be encountered in handling, transporting, and disposing of the solid waste is essential. People picking up such material should be aware of the hazards and informed of what to do in case of a spill during transport.

The solid chemical wastes of a laboratory should be placed into containers provided for that purpose. When bottles are used, they should be placed in carriers. All wastes must be adequately labeled. The laboratory worker should be aware of the hazards that may be involved in disposing of particular solid chemical wastes and the importance of segregating incompatible materials.

Liquid Chemical Wastes

As with solid chemical wastes, each organization should have a procedure for collecting liquid chemical wastes from its laboratories and arranging for their disposal. Suitable containers should be provided, and the laboratory workers should understand what may or may not be placed in these containers and which materials require special labeling.

Waste solvents that are free of solids and corrosive or reactive substances may be collected in a common bottle or can, which is taken away when full. If this system is used, it is essential to consider exactly what mixtures, which may include waste from another laboratory, will go into the can and whether the substances involved are compatible.

Segregation into two or three types of waste is often useful (*e.g.,* chlorinated solvents, hydrocarbons), as is the use of completely separate bottles for waste that poses special difficulties. Chlorinated solvents form hydrogen chloride on combustion and must be segregated from materials destined for incineration. Separated and well-defined waste is easier to discard. All hazardous waste must be so labeled.

Some solvents (*e.g.,* ethers and secondary alcohols) form explosive peroxides on standing. Some reactions can cause explosions directly (*e.g., acetone plus chloroform in the presence of a base*). Others, such as acid–base interactions, can generate sufficient heat to vaporize or ignite flammable materials such as carbon disulfide. The addition of hot materials can cause the buildup of pressure in a tightly closed solvent container, with the potential for compressive ignition. The acid formed when halogenated solvents are left moist can corrode cans, as can any dissolved corrosive in a discarded mixture.

When large quantities of a solvent are involved, consideration should be given to recycling rather than disposal, although this operation also involves some potential hazards and expense.

Hazardous Wastes

Hazardous wastes include very toxic substances, strong carcinogens, mutagens, and explosives. The laboratory worker has a responsibility to ensure that proper arrangements for disposal of these materials are made. Wherever possible, chemical procedures to produce less hazardous substances should be undertaken. In the case of chemicals regulated as carcinogens, EPA disposal rules must be followed. A spill of a hazardous substance can be an especially serious hazard. Personnel working with such substances should have emergency plans.

Nonhazardous Wastes

Nonhazardous waste, depending on its physical state, may be flushed into a laboratory sink or exhausted slowly in an operating fume hood.

If the waste is in the solid state and there is no danger of its reacting with other common waste, it may be discarded in a noncombustible waste container.

Chemical Disposal Methods

- Collect flammable liquids in suitable containers for disposal.
- A metal safety container with a self-closing cover for disposal of pledgets and solvent-soaked swabs prevents release and possible ignition of flammable vapors.
- Broken glassware and disposable syringes should be deposited in separate, labeled containers. Separation helps to prevent injury in handling regular waste and to ensure proper final disposal if these materials are disposed of separately.
- Acidic and alkaline wastes should be neutralized prior to being introduced into the sewer system.
- Safety containers should be provided for the collection of flammable wastes; such waste should not be deposited in the sewer system. Some flammable wastes and many other chemicals may be neutralized if the quantities are not too large.
- When combustibles are burned in incinerators, particular care should be taken to prevent aerosol cans from being disposed of

with the combustibles. The explosive force of such cans, when heated, may cause a blowback, striking the incinerator operator.

- Miscellaneous waste (*i.e.,* metal containers, bottles, broken glassware, ether cans, aerosol cans, light bulbs, fluorescent tubes, and other noncombustible trash) should be discarded in specially designated waste receptacles.

- Disposal of solid chemicals (*e.g.,* sodium, potassium, calcium carbide, phosphoric anhydride, and phosphorus) and more than 1-liter quantities of such liquids as thionyl chloride and phosphorus oxychloride should be handled by a qualified disposal technician.

- Mercaptans should never be poured down the drain. Chemicals that may create highly toxic fumes when they come into contact with other chemicals in the drain system should be discarded in containers.

- Some chemicals can be destroyed by other chemicals before being discarded (*e.g.,* sodium by ethanol, potassium by tertiary butyl alcohol). This requires expert advice and supervision.

- To prevent water from splashing into the bottle and causing a violent reaction, extreme care must be taken in the disposal of fuming or concentrated sulfuric acid. When quantities exceeding 0.5 liter are to be discarded, the waste liquid should be transferred into the empty original bottle by means of a dipper and funnel; the bottle should then be removed from the building.

Radioactive-Waste Disposal*

Radioactive waste from RIA procedures is waste of very low-level radioactivity. Liquids from RIA testing may safely be poured into a sink and flushed well with water. Absorbent paper and solid waste from RIA kits may be discarded with routine trash *after* radioactive labels are removed. RIA waste may be kept for several days before disposal, under conditions approved by the radiation safety officer, in a properly shielded container while the radioactivity decays. As previously mentioned, even radioactivity at these reduced levels may be regulated in

---

*This section refers to only that radioactive waste from RIA procedures. It does not apply to waste from nuclear medicine.

some jurisdictions. If that is the case, special labeling, pickup, and removal may be required for all RIA waste (Fig. 9-6). This may include liquids as well.

"Safe" Paper Waste

Nonhazardous waste, including paper, paper towels, scrap paper, and other generally safe waste may be disposed of in routine trash. This waste should be segregated as it is generated and may be collected and disposed of by housekeeping personnel in accordance with hospital policy. Carelessly combining this waste in with more hazardous waste generally adds to costs and must be avoided.

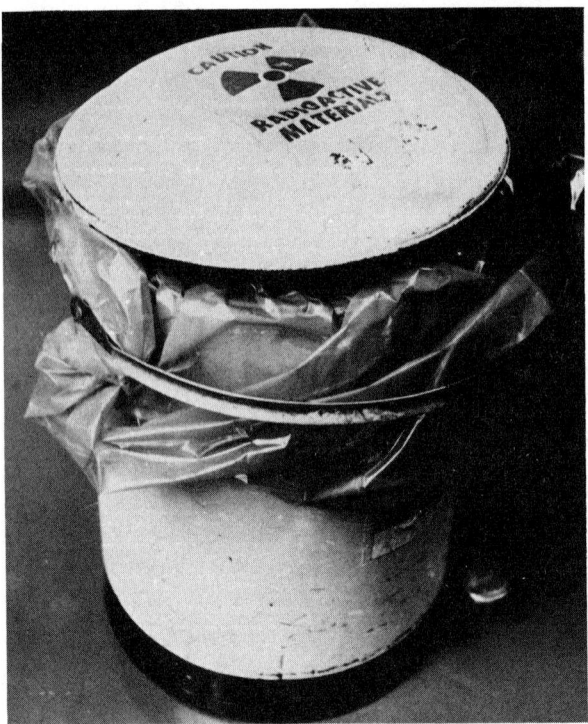

Fig. 9-6. When regulations dictate, special well-marked containers are required for disposal of materials used in RIA tests.

Appendix A
OSHA General Industry Standards

**SUBJECT INDEX FOR OSHA SAFETY AND
HEALTH STANDARDS
TITLE 29 CFR, PART 1910**

Subparts

    A* —General
    B* —Adoptional Extension of Established Federal Standards
    C   —Reserved
    D* —Walking and Working Surfaces
    E* —Means of Egress
    F   —Powered Platforms, Manlifts and Vehicle Mounted Work Platforms
    G* —Occupational Health and Environmental Control
    H* —Hazardous Materials
    I* —Personal Protective Equipment
    J* —General Environmental Controls
    K* —Medical and First Aid
    L* —Fire Protection
    M* —Compressed Gas and Compressed Air Equipment

N —Materials Handling and Storage
O —Machinery and Machine Guarding
P —Hand and Portable Powered Tools and Other Hand Held Equipment
Q —Welding, Cutting, Brazing
R —Special Industries
S* —Electrical
T —Commercial Driving Operations
U–Y—Reserved
Z* —Toxic and Hazardous Substances

*Subparts relevant to the clinical laboratory worker

Subpart Z—Toxic and Hazardous Substances—Current Status and Contents

- *1910·1000 Air Contaminant Tables Z-1, Z-2, Z-3*

These tables list several hundred air contaminants to which employees may be exposed. They stipulate permissible exposure limits (PELs) for each regulated chemical. These limits are *legally* enforceable in the clinical laboratory. Owing to the unique conditions in the laboratory, however, measurement and monitoring of these substances may present a problem because the levels of exposure are so low. Newer laboratory methods attempt to avoid use of these chemicals whenever and wherever safer substances may be substituted.

- *1910·1001–1910·1045 OSHA-Regulated High-Risk Chemicals*

Currently, OSHA carcinogen standards and other high-risk chemical standards stand as valuable guidelines for the clinical laboratory in handling these substances. Compliance is *recommended* but not presently *legally required.* These standards were designed for the industrial workplace and some of the requirements (*e.g.,* showers, changing rooms, environmental monitoring) are therefore not appropriate to the clinical laboratory. In industry these requirements are primarily met through engineering and environmental controls, while the small amounts of such chemicals that may be found in the clinical laboratory can be handled safely with personal-protection devices-gloves, fume hoods, restricted-use areas, and so on.

In the event that this regulatory situation is modified to address specifically the laboratory setting (research, clinical, or academic), the PELs will remain intact, but the requirements for exposure to high-risk chemicals will be tailored to the laboratory use of these chemicals. Notification of this regulatory change, when it occurs, will be communicated by OSHA in the *Federal*

Register, clinical-laboratory professional journals, newsletters, and other widely distributed publications.

Single-Substance Standards

Asbestos
Vinyl chloride
Inorganic arsenic
Lead
1,2-dibromo-3-chloropropane
Acrylonitrile

Carcinogens

alpha-Naphthylamine
Methyl chloromethyl ether
3,3′-Dichlorobenzidine and its salts
bis-Chloromethyl ether
beta-Naphthylamine
Benzidine
4-Aminodiphenyl
Ethyleneimine
beta-Propiolactone
2-acetylaminofluorene
4-Dimethylaminoazobenzene
N-Nitrosodimethylamine
4-Nitrobiphenyl

Appendix B
Accreditation Standards

Accreditation standards for medical laboratories have been established by the College of American Pathologists (CAP), the Joint Commission on Accreditation for Hospitals (JCAH), and the American Osteopathic Association (AOA). Excerpts from the 1983 CAP standards are presented here to illustrate the format of the standards. In the full text, each standard is followed by an interpretation and explanatory notes. Similar format and approach are used by all three accrediting bodies. Notice the very general level at which the standards are written. The actual on-site inspection by the accrediting agency uses a very detailed checklist based on these general standards. The checklist itself is available to the laboratory before the inspection so that a satisfactory level of safety can be attained.

STANDARDS FOR LABORATORY ACCREDITATION*

Standard I

The practice of pathology is essential to patient care. The pathologist and the laboratory staff shall provide appropriate services, including, but not limited to, the examination of patient related specimens, clinical interpretation

*Excerpted with permission of the College of American Pathologists, Skokie, IL.

and consultation, scientific investigation, and education in order to be effective in the prevention, recognition, diagnosis, treatment, and prognosis of disease.

Standard II

The laboratories shall have sufficient space, equipment, facilities, and supplies for the performance of the required volume of work with accuracy, precision, efficiency, and safety: in addition, the laboratories shall have methods for communication to ensure prompt, reliable reporting and appropriate record storage and retrieval.

Interpretation

The scope of the responsibilities and activities of the laboratory must be delineated. Once this determination has been made, sufficient space, equipment, and qualified personnel must be provided.

The environment within the laboratory shall be conducive to effective performance of personnel and equipment. Work assignments shall be consistent with the qualifications of the technical personnel. There shall be sufficient, conveniently located bench and storage space for the proper handling of specimens and housing of equipment and reagents. Special areas for tests requiring a controlled environment shall be provided. Work areas shall be arranged to minimize transportation and communication problems, and shall be adequately lighted to facilitate performance of analytical procedures . . .

Facilities, equipment, and instruments shall be appropriate for the services performed and must be maintained in a demonstrably functional condition.

The laboratory must be a safe working place for the personnel and for the patients it serves. The laboratory must be in compliance with the relevant safety codes of the appropriate jurisdictional authority and of the federal government. The safe handling of patient samples and of reagents shall be an integral part of the laboratory safety program. Proper disposal of hazardous wastes shall be provided.

Standard III

A hospital pathology service shall be directed by a physician who is an active member of the medical staff and is qualified to assume professional, organizational, educational, and administrative responsibility for the service. The director of an independent laboratory shall be a physician with training and experience in pathology, or a clinical scientist with adequate training and experience in clinical laboratory work, who meets the requirements of a laboratory director under the Clinical Laboratory Improvement Act of 1967. The director shall be responsible for ensuring that there are sufficient personnel with adequate training and experience to supervise and conduct the work of the pathology service.

Standard IV

Each laboratory, whether a hospital or independent laboratory, shall have a quality control system designed to assure the reliability and medical usefulness of laboratory data.

Interpretation

. . . The laboratory shall submit to periodic inspection and evaluation as determined by the Commission on Laboratory Accreditation of the College of American Pathologists.

ACCREDITING AGENCY ADDRESSES

To obtain the complete text of standards for each of the three accrediting agencies, write to the following:

Standards for Accreditation of Medical Laboratories
    College of American Pathologists
    7400 North Skokie Boulevard
    Skokie, Illinois 60077

JCAH Accreditation Manual for Hospitals
    Joint Commission on Accreditation for Hospitals—Publications
    875 North Michigan Avenue
    Chicago, Illinois 60611

Requirements and Interpretive Guide for Accredited Hospitals of the American Osteopathic Association
    American Osteopathic Association
    212 East Ohio Street
    Chicago, Illinois 60611

Appendix C
College of American Pathologists' Laboratory Checklist

Accreditation standards form the basis for the detailed checklists used by the site-visit team on the inspection visit to the laboratory. These checklists are available to the laboratory *before* the visit.

The following is excerpted from the 1983 CAP checklist and contains only the safety-related portions.* In the CAP checklist, safety sections appear in both the Laboratory General Section *and* in the section for each separate laboratory. Sections reproduced here are from Laboratory General, Chemistry, Hematology, and Nuclear Medicine In-vitro Procedures.

LABORATORY GENERAL

Laboratory Safety

Questions in this section will cover the General Safety Program for the entire laboratory and must be answered for all laboratories. Specific questions related to safety features peculiar to an individual section will be found in the checklist for that section.

---

*Excerpted with permission of the College of American Pathologists, Skokie, IL.

Policies and Procedures

It is strongly recommended that a laboratory safety manual be developed to define specific policies and procedures for the entire laboratory.

Are safety policies and procedures written and adequate?

Are safety policies and procedures posted or readily available to all personnel?

Have policies and procedures been developed regarding the documentation and reporting of laboratory incidents and accidents?

Does the safety manual include sections, as appropriate, for the laboratory relating to

General requirements for personnel and laboratory safety?

Fire prevention and control?

Electrical safety?

Compressed gases?

Chemical and toxic hazards?

Carcinogens?

Microbiologic hazards?

Hazardous waste disposal?

Internal and external disaster plans?

Does the laboratory have a designated safety officer or representative(s)?

Fire Safety

Is the laboratory separated from surrounding hospital areas and from exit corridors by fire resistant construction with a minimum rating of one hour and with C-label doors?

Note—A C-label door is of fire resistive construction and has a rating of 3/4 of an hour.

Are fire drills held periodically?

Are fire escape routes (fire exits) convenient to the laboratory?

Are evacuation routes diagrammed and posted?

Do all rooms in which major hazards exist have direct access to the hall or a second exit?

Is the fire bell, PA system, or other fire alarm system audible in all sections of the laboratory?

Is there a fire alarm station in or near the laboratory?

Note—Some instructions and/or buildings may use a telephone network as a fire alarm system and this is acceptable.

Is smoking prohibited in all technical work areas?

Are there sufficient fire extinguishers (CO_2 and dry chemical) and fire blankets in the department?

Have personnel been instructed in the use of fire extinguishers and fire blankets?

Are safety cans used for appropriate volumes of highly volatile liquids such as ether?

Note—Small volumes (one pint or less) of highly volatile liquids in current use may be stored on open shelves. The small, plastic-stoppered, tin cans used for shipment and supply of ether are considered safety cans.

Are bulk supplies of flammable liquids properly stored (*i.e.,* in a safety room or cabinet)?

Is the amount of flammable liquids in any safety cabinet less than 60 gallons per 5000 square feet of laboratory area?

Are storage areas and/or rooms where volatile solvents are used adequately ventilated?

Are flammable or combustible liquids or gas cylinders positioned well away from open flame or other heat sources, not in corridors and not within exhaust canopies?

Is there evidence of the capacity to ground a secondary container when flammables are decanted from large drum (bulk) containers?

Are flammable gas cylinders stored in a separate ventilated room or enclosure reserved exclusively for that purpose; and which has a fire resistance classification of at least 1 hour?

Is an emergency water supply (shower or hose flushing device) convenient to areas where caustic materials are used (reagent preparation, acid cleaning of glassware, and other high risk areas)?

Have personnel been instructed in the safe handling of corrosive and caustic materials (i.e., handle only one bottle at a time, use of carts or carriers for transporting) and use of transfer devices and safety procedures?

Are acid bottle carriers used for all large containers (over 500 ml) of caustic and corrosive materials?

Are explicit instructions posted for the emergency treatment of acid splashes and injuries and the control of acid spills?

Is a handtruck used for transporting gas cylinders and are the cylinders properly secured to the truck?

Is emergency lighting adequate for safe evacuation available in the laboratory?

Electrical Safety

Are electrical outlets periodically checked for ground integrity?

Are there records of checks for ground integrity of electrical outlets?

Have all personnel been instructed as to shock hazards, precautions, and emergency procedures?

Toxic and Biologic Hazards

The basic requirements for safety from toxic or biologic hazards include proper notification of personnel (area posted, labels attached, etc.), identification of the type of hazard (poison, caustics, skin or eye irritant), precautions to be taken to avoid hazard, and instructions about what to do if accidental exposure or contamination does occur. Additional requirements for dangerous materials (such as carcinogens) include having a valid use permit, controlling access to the area, and monitoring personnel. The laboratory should conduct an inventory of all materials listed as hazardous or carcinogenic by OSHA to avoid penalties for non-compliance.

Have known potential toxic and biologic hazards in the laboratory been defined and policies established to minimize their danger?

Hepatitis infection is a laboratory hazard. Specimens from patients suspected or known to have hepatitis should be labeled in a distinctive manner, handled and disposed of in a manner that minimizes the hazard.

Are specimens from patients suspected of hepatitis identified and labeled in a distinctive manner?

Is the distinctive label retained by the specimen or subdivisions of the specimen as it travels through the laboratory?

Have policies been established and technologists instructed in the proper handling of suspected hepatitis specimens?

Are eating and drinking prohibited in the technical work areas?

Is the application of cosmetics prohibited in the technical work areas?

Is mouth pipetting prohibited in all areas of the laboratory?

Note—Mechanical pipetting devices should be available and used.

Are vacuum breakers (anti-siphon devices) provided on water outlets where necessary?

Note—Necessary only if the spigot or an extension extends below sink level or if the outlet has a suction apparatus attached.

OSHA has promulgated standards for exposure, to chemicals considered to be carcinogenic (*i.e.,* Class I carcinogens).* Their listing includes the following:

4-Nitrobiphenyl
4,4-methylene bis (2-chloraniline)
3,3'-Dichlorobenzidine
beta-Naphthylamine
4-Aminodiphenyl

*U.S. Code of Federal Regulations 45, No. 157, 1980

beta-Propiolactone
4-Dimethylaminoazobenzene
Vinyl chloride
alpha-Naphthylamine
Methyl chloromethyl ether
bis-Chloromethyl ether
Benzidine
Ethyleneimine
2-acetylaminofluorene
N-Nitrosodimethylamine
Benzene

Has the laboratory been inventoried for the presence of confirmed
    (Class I) carcinogens?

If carcinogens and/or suspected carcinogens are used in the labora-
    tory, have these been properly identified and policies established
    for their safe handling, use, and disposal?

Waste Disposal

The laboratory is responsible for real or potential hazards of wastes at all
stages of disposal including transportation and final disposition. Prevailing
local, state, and federal (EPA) regulations should be reviewed by the
Laboratory Director, Safety Officer, or hospital engineer to be sure that the
laboratory is in compliance with regulations.

Is the method for disposal of all solid and liquid wastes in compliance
    with local, state, and federal regulations?

Are solid wastes such as discarded glassware, blood collection tubes,
    specimens, and bacteriologic wastes safely disposed of?
    Note—1) Contaminated material should be disinfected prior to dis-
    carding; 2) contaminated material should be burned or buried
    (i.e., not end up in an open dump); 3) contaminated material
    should be double bagged and properly marked to indicate the
    type of hazard and whom to notify if breakage or leakage occurs
    prior to final disposal. (Laboratory Safety at the CDC 75-8118)

Is broken glass discarded in a properly marked and safe container?

Are disposable needles and syringes destroyed and discarded in a safe
    manner (separate container, adequately marked to avoid injury to
    custodial personnel)?

CHEMISTRY

Are items of protective clothing (aprons, heat resistant gloves,
    rubber gloves, goggles, face shields) available in areas where
    indicated?

Have personnel been instructed in the proper use of protective clothing?

Is the heating of flammable liquids performed only in a suitable fume hood and utilizing acceptable heat sources?

Is the supply of compressed gases being held for immediate use within the laboratory, no more than two days' working supply or one minimally sized container of each gas?

Are gas cylinders secured in accordance with safety standards?

Is the proper regulator used for the gas in question? The use of adaptors should be prohibited.

Are acetylene cylinders properly piped, tanks chained to the wall and handled according to established procedures? (Should comply with NFPA 51 Standard for the Operation of Oxygen-Fuel Gas Systems.)

Does the acetylene tank or line have a safety shut-off valve?

Are known toxic, caustic, and other hazardous materials adequately labeled?

Is an emergency water supply (shower or hose flushing device) convenient to areas where caustic materials are used (reagent preparation, acid cleaning of glassware, and other high risk areas)?

Have personnel been instructed in the safe handling of corrosive and caustic materials (*i.e.,* handle only one bottle at a time, use carts or carriers for transporting) and use of transfer devices and safety procedures?

Are acid bottle carriers used for all large containers (over 500 ml)?

Electrical Safety

Are all instruments adequately grounded and checked periodically? Note—As a general rule, this refers to instruments with metal cases. Instruments with plastic cases (such as microscopes) may not need to be grounded.

Are policies and procedures developed for the safe handling of electrophoretic equipment?

Biologic Hazards

Have policies been established and technologists thoroughly instructed in the proper handling of suspected hepatitis specimens?

Have all clinical chemistry personnel been instructed concerning the potential hazards of aerosols produced by centrifugation of biologic specimens?

HEMATOLOGY

Diluents for automatic cell counters may contain low concentrations of sodium azides as a preservative. Sodium azide, when disposed of into lead or copper pipes, or into plumbing with lead packed joints, may form insoluble and highly explosive azide salts.

Are "azide *free*" reagents used with automated cell counters?

(If "YES," this checklist is complete; if "NO," complete next four questions.)

If azide containing solutions are emptied into lead or copper pipes, is there a written procedure for the safe disposal of this material (*i.e.,* flushing, etc.)?

Is the procedure for proper disposal of azides regularly followed?

If a potential hazard exists (azide solutions in lead or copper lines), has a notice been posted to warn persons working on lines of the potential danger and to avoid work on pipe joints?

Are methods available for cleaning insoluble azide salts from pipes when indicated?

NUCLEAR MEDICINE IN-VITRO PROCEDURES

Is there a radiation safety manual?

Is the manual updated as new policies or procedures are introduced?

Does the radiation safety manual include a section on decontamination?

Are there specific policies regarding authorization or restriction of personnel handling radionuclides?

Are there written procedures for handling spills?

Are there written procedures for handling radioactive waste?

Do policies include procedures for inspection, monitoring of shipment, and notification in the event of a damaged or leaking radionuclide shipment?

Are shipments of radionuclides delivered directly to the RIA lab and not left unattended?

Are all shipments of radionuclides logged?

Are all areas or rooms where radioactive materials are being used or stored posted to indicate the presence of radioactive materials?

Are radionuclide storage and decay areas properly shielded?

Are radionuclide storage and decay areas locked when not under the supervision of lab personnel?

Is radioactive trash (syringes, alcohol wipes) kept separate from normal trash?

Are all personnel instructed in the use of radiation monitoring devices?

Are all technical personnel instructed in decontamination routines?

Are all personnel instructed in the safe handling and proper disposal of radionuclides (syringes, needles, and sponges)?

Is there a portable survey meter?

Are survey instruments calibrated regularly?

Are there regular radiation area surveys and wipe tests with records maintained?

Are tolerance limits established for each area surveyed and wiped?

Are work benches and sinks decontaminated each day of use?

Is there evidence that a laboratory representative is a member of and/or attends the radiation safety committee regularly?

Note—This question N/A for independent (non-hospital) laboratories (see next question).

Does the laboratory have a radiation safety officer who is responsible for and actively monitors radiation safety?

Note—Primarily applicable to independent (non-hospital) laboratories, but may be appropriate for laboratories in very large institutions.

Appendix D
Reagents Used in
Some Common Procedures

The following section lists some significant reagents that are required in the performance of some common clinical laboratory test procedures. This list was culled from the procedures manual of a large urban clinical hospital laboratory. The language and abbreviations are provided here as they appear in the original manual.

The purpose of this appendix is to bring to your attention the serious nature of some of the substances with which you work, as well as to illustrate the very incomplete nature of the information generally provided to the laboratory staff. Often this appendix lists reagents only by letter, number, or trade name, or calls them only "reagent" or "stain." In most cases, of course, all the constituent chemicals are listed. This appendix intends not to be complete or to provide all the information required to perform a test, but rather to identify some hazardous chemicals and to encourage the reading of *all* labels and warnings on reagent containers.

Availability of complete information on all chemicals encountered is a valid goal for the clinical laboratory and may be legally required under the right-to-know laws in some states. (See Chaps. 1 and 3.)

Chemistry

TEST	REAGENT
Total and prostatic acid phosphatase	Citrate buffer (citric acid monohydrate)
	Sodium hydroxide 1N
	Hydrochloric acid 0.1N
	Tartrate citrate buffer
	Tartaric acid
	Citrate buffer
	Substrate
	p-nitrophenyl
Alkaline phosphatase	*p*-nitrophenyl/phosphate
	Magnesium chloride 1M
	Sodium hydroxide 0.02N
Amylase	Cibachron blue (a monochloratriazine dye)
Barbiturates	Chloroform
	Phosphate solution
	Phosphate buffer
	Ammonium chloride
	Hydrochloric acid 0.1N
Bilirubin	Sulfanilic acid
	Sodium nitrite
	Diazo—Sodium nitrite and sulfuric acid
	Fehling's reagent
	Hydrochloric acid 0.05N
BSP	Bromsulphalein dye
Calcium	Potassium hydroxide 1N
	Potassium chloride
Carotene	95% ethanol
	Potassium dichromate
	Petroleum ether
Calculus analysis	Hydrochloric acid 1.65 M (eye irritant)
	Manganese dioxide (eye irritant)
	Hydrochloric acid
	Mercuric iodide
	Potassium iodide
	Sodium cyanide (*poison*)
	Sodium hydroxide 2M (*poison*)

	p-Nitrobenzeneazoresorcinol
	Sodium hydroxide
	Ammonium molybdate
	Ferrous ammonium sulfate (eye irritant)
	Sulfuric acid
	Calcein
	Potassium hydroxide
	Neocuproine
	Copper sulfate
	Acetic acid
	Sodium nitroferricyanide (*poison*)
	Chloroform
Chloride/CO_2 analyzer	Potassium chloride
	Potassium bicarbonate
	Sulfuric acid
γ-GT	Gamma-glutamyl transpeptidase
	Nitroanilide derivatives (hazardous if ingested or absorbed)
Glycosylated hemoglobulin test AIC	Elution/developing reagent (*poison*, should not be pipetted by mouth)
HDL cholesterol	Phosphotungstic acid
Hemoglobin electrophoresis	Trichloroacetic acid
	Methanol
	Glacial acetic acid
Hemoglobin F by alkali denaturation	Potassium hydroxide 3.5N (20%)
	Ammonium sulfate (acidified)
LDH isozymes on cellulose acetate	Nitroblue tetrazoleum
	Phenazine methasulfate
Total lipid	Sulfuric acid
ROPES test—examination of mucin	Acetic acid
	Hyaluronic acid
Serum protein electrophoresis	Glacial acetic acid
	Trichloroacetic acid
	Methanol
	Ethanol
Urine and CSF protein	Coomassie brilliant blue G250 dye (corrosive; do not pipette by mouth)

Salicylate

Nitric Acid 0.07N
Ferric nitrate
Salicylic acid
Chloroform

Foam stability test (modified elements)

Shake test (CFS)

Absolute ethanol (100%)

Urea nitrogen manual

All reagents harmful if swallowed

Uric acid

Uric acid
Cupric reagent

Xylose absorption procedure

p-bromoaniline
Glacial acetic acid

Ethyl alcohol

Ethanol
Trichloroacetic acid

Acetaminophen (Tylenol)

Orthocresol
4M—ammonium hydroxide
5% trichloroacetic acid

Colorimetric preg-estrogens

Ethyl acetate
Sulfuric Acid
Hydroquinone
Trichloroacetic acid—do not pipette by mouth
Chloroform—harmful vapor
Hydrochloric acid
Ethyl alcohol

VMA—24-hr urine

Vanillylmandelic acid
Ethyl acetate
Diazotized p-nitroaniline
Hydrochloric acid buffer
Tetrabutylammonium hydroxide
Ethyl acetate/ethanol
Glacial acetic acid
Diazo reagent
    Sodium nitrite (*highly toxic*)
    p-nitroaniline

Chemistry Stat Lab

TEST	REAGENT
Ethyl alcohol level	Nicotinamide-adenine dinucleotide (NAD) alcohol dehydrogenase (ADH) Ethanol solution Pyrophosphate buffer Trichloroacetic acid
Blood ammonia	Ammonia reagent (α-ketoglutarate and NADH) L-Glutamic dehydrogenase (GLDH) Ammonia control
Bilirubin	Caffeine Sulfanilic acid Sodium nitrite Diazo (sodium nitrite and sulfanilic acid) Stabilizer Fehling's reagent Hydrochloric acid 0.05N
Calcium	Cresolphtalein complex one Diethylamine
Chloride	Nitric acetic reagent PVA H_2O + powdered polyvinyl alcohol Sodium chloride
Blood ketone	Buffers Glycine nitroprusside
Magnesium	Magnesium dye reagent Magnesium base reagent Magnesium reference standard
Spinal fluid protein	Magnesium iodate Hydrochloric acid Trichloroacetic acid Sodium chloride

Salicylate   Nitric acid
                                    Ferric nitrate
                                    Salicylic acid
                                    Chloroform

Urinalysis

TEST	REAGENT
Phenylketonuria	Sulfuric acid 6N 10% ferric chloride
Serial dilution for tryspin activity	Barbital buffer (sodium diethylbarbiturate) X-ray film, undeveloped
Sudan IV fat stain	95% ethanol Sudan IV
VMA 24-hr urine	Strong acid preservative in collection bottle: careful
Carcinoid (serotonin)	1-nitroso-2-naphthol Nitrous acid (sodium nitrite + sulfuric acid 2N) Ethylene dichloride
Glucose tolerance	Clinitest tablets Acetest tablets Clinistix
Bence Jones protein	Sulfosalicylic acid
Urine + CSF protein	Coomassie brilliant blue dye Stabilizer—methanol
Quantitative urobilinogen in urine	Ehrlich's reagent Paradiethylamine benzaldehyde Hydrochloric acid Water Sodium acetate
Protein	Sulfosalicyclic acid
Bile pigments + derivatives	Bichloride of mercury
Fat in urine	Ether
Quantitative bilirubin in urine	95% ethanol

	Concentrated hydrochloric acid Diazo reagent Sodium nitrite
Fecal urobilinogen and urobilin	Ethanol Zinc acetate Sodium acetate Ehrlich's reagent
Diacetic acid	Acetoacetic acid 10% ferric chloride
Myoglobin	Ammonium sulfate
Reducing substances in stool	Hydrochloric acid 1N
Porphyrin	Glacial acetic acid Hydrochloric acid Talc
Porphobilinogen	Ehrlich's reagent, modified Hydrochloric acid Paradimethylamine benzaldehyde Water Zinc acetate Chloroform
pH	Methyl red Bromthymol blue
Protein	Tetrabromphenol blue
Glucose	Glucose oxidase Peroxidase Potassium iodide
Ketones	Sodium nitroprusside
Bilirubin	2,4-dichloroaniline diazonium salt
Blood	Cumene hydroperoxide Orthotolidine
Nitrite	Para-arsanilic acid N-(1-napthyl) ethylenediamine dihydro- chloride
Urobilinogen	Paradimethylamine-benzaldehyde

Hematology

TEST	REAGENT
QC for Coulter S	Clorox clean aperture (or other detergent)
Coulter	Isoton buffered saline
Reticulocyte stain	Methylene blue Oxalate Methyl violet Sodium chloride
G6PD	Trisma buffer
Eosonophil count	Propylene glycol Distilled water Phloxine Sodium bicarbonate
Spinal fluid cell counts	Glacial acetic acid Alcoholic gentian violet Distilled water
Sickledex	Sickledex powder buffer
Free HGB	Hematest tablet

Bone marrow iron stain	Iron stain
	Vapor formal ethanol (vapor 10 ml, 40%
	  formaldehyde)
	Potassium ferrocyanide
	Nuclear fast red stain (nuclear fast red
	  aluminum sulfate)
	Hydrochloric acid

Hemoglobin F	McElvaine's buffer Citric acid Dibasic sodium phosphate
Stains	Giemsa Wright's

Leukocyte alkaline phosphatase
  stain kit
	Fixative
	  10% formalin in absolute methanol
	  Citrate buffered acetone
	Stain
	  Naphthol AS-MX phosphate concentrate

Fast blue
Fast red
Mayer's hematoxylin
Manganese chloride
Glycerol gelatin

Gugol stain   Catalyst
Reagent
Acetone free reagent grade methyl alcohol

Carboxyhemoglobin   20% Sodium hydroxide
10% ammonium sulfide

Acid serum test of PNH   Hydrochloric acid 1/5N

Prussian blue   10% Potassium ferrocyanide

Urine sediment   20% Hydrochloric acid

Heinz bodies   Methyl violet

Heinz body   Acetylphenylhydrazine
Crystal violet
Sodium chloride

Maternal from newborn blood   Saline
(in vomit, stool)   1% sodium chloride

Autohemolysis   Sodium chloride

G6PD spot test   Sodium ascorbate
Sodium cyanide
Hydrochloric acid 2N
Isotonic phosphate buffer
    NaH_2PO_4, H_2O
    Na_2HPO_4

G6PD DEAE cellulose   Tris HCl, .01% potassium cyanide

Unstable hemoglobin   Isopropanol solution
Concentrated hydrochloric acid

Hema-tek stainer

Isopropanol precipitation   10% isopropyl alcohol
Concentrated hydrochloric acid

	Carbon tetrachloride
	2% potassium cyanide
Inclusion bodies	Citrate saline
(HgbH)	Sodium citrate
	Brilliant cresyl blue
Hemostasis testing	Almost all alike; a salt (*e.g.,* calcium chloride); little else
Plasma protime	Sodium citrate
Plasma recalcifracation time	Sodium citrate
	Calcium chloride
Factor identification testing	
Fibrin stabilizing factor	Calcium chloride
	Urea solution
Factor assay	Activated cephaloplastin
	Calcium chloride
	Owen's veronal buffer

Microbiology

TEST	REAGENT

General

API test for enterobacteriaceae	Kovac's reagent
	Hydrochloric acid
	n-amyl alcohol
	Paradimethylaminebenzaldehyde
	Ferric chloride
	VP reagents
	Absolute alcohol
	Alphanaphthol
	Potassium hydroxide
	Nitrate reduction reagents
	Acetic acid
	Sulfanilic acid
	N,N-dimethyl-alpha-naphthylamine
	Oxidase test
	N,N,N^1,N^1-tetramethyl-*p*-phenylene-diamine
	Dihydrochloride
Culture media examples	Nitrate broth
	Sulfanilic acid

Zinc dust
Dimethyl alpha-napthylamine
Tryptone for idol
Xylene
Ehrlich's reagent
Oxidase test
Tetramethyl paraphenylene diamine di-
hydrochloride

BACT-CHEK

Viable organisms

Gram's stain

Crystal violet
Gram's iodine
Ethanol
Acetone
Safranin

Parasitology

Permanent stain from PVA
preserved material

10% formalin
Alcohol
Acetic acid
Xylene

Formalin ether concentration
method

Formalin
Ether

Trichrome stain

Modified Schaudinn's fixative
Schaudinn's fixative
Ethyl alcohol
Mercuric chloride
Alcohol/iodine
Acid/alcohol
Carbol-xylene
Xylene
Trichrome stain
Chromotrope, phosphotungstic acid
Light green
Fast green
Glacial acetic acid

Lawless rapid permanent mount
stain for protozoa

Acetone
Glacial acetic acid
Formaldehyde

Schaudinn's solution
Acid fuchsin
Fast green FCF
Xylol

Stool exam for parasites and formed elements

Concentration in ethyl ether

PVA—preserved fecal suspensions

Ethyl alcohol
Iodine
Modified Schaudinn's fixture
   Glacial acetic acid
   Glycerol
   Ethyl alcohol
   Mercuric chloride

MIF stain—preservation technique for intestinal protozoa

Thimerosal
Formaldehyde
Lugol's iodine

Mycology

Ziehl-Neelsen staining method for TB

Carbolfuchsin stain
   Basic fuchsin
   Ethanol
Phenol

Hydrochloric acid

Acid alcohol
Hydrochloric acid
Ethanol
Methylene blue

Sputum concentration for TB

N-acetyl-1-cysteine — hydrochloric acid
Benzalkonium chloride

Fluorescent and acid-fast double staining for mycobacteria

Truant's fluorescent dye
   Auramine O
   Rhodamine B
   Glycerol
   Phenol
   Acid alcohol
   Acid-fast stain
      Kinyoun's carbol fuschin
         Basic fuchsin
         Phenol
   Acid alcohol

Alcohol
Hydrochloric acid
Methylene blue
Ethyl alcohol

Blood Bank/Serology/Radioimmunoassay

TEST	REAGENT
Blood bank	All reagents contain sodium azide as a preservative, 1:100
Colloidal gold (serology)	Gold chloride Sodium citrate Hydrogen peroxide
Radioimmunoassay	1 radioactive tracer per test
Hepatitis-associated antigen	Positive control serum HAA-specific antibody

Appendix E
Resources for
Safety Information

PROFESSIONAL SOCIETIES AND ORGANIZATIONS

American Medical Association (AMA)
535 N. Dearborn Avenue
Chicago, Illinois 60610

American Society for Medical Technology (ASMT)
1725 DeSales
Suite 403
Washington, D.C. 20036
also
330 Meadowfern Drive
Houston, Texas 77067

Armed Forces Institute of Pathology
6825 16th Street, N.W.
Washington, D.C. 20306

American Society for Clinical Chemistry
1725 K Street, N.W.
Washington, D.C. 20036

American Society for Microbiology
1913 I Street, N.W.
Washington, D.C. 20006

American Board of Pathology
112 Lincoln Center
5401 West Kennedy Boulevard
Tampa, Florida 33623

American College of Physicians
4200 Pine Street
Philadelphia, Pennsylvania 19104

Association of American Medical Colleges
One DuPont Circle
Washington, D.C. 20036

American Hospital Association (AHA)
444 North Capitol Street, N.W.
Suite 500
Washington, D.D. 20001

American Public Health Association (APHA)
1015 15th Street, N.W.
Washington, D.C. 20005

Underwriters Laboratories, Inc.
333 Pfingsten Road
Northbrook, Illinois 60662

American National Standards Institute
1430 Broadway
New York, New York 10018

National Commission for Laboratory Standards and Guidelines
771 Lancaster Avenue
Villanova, Pennsylvania 19085

College of American Pathology (CAP)
1101 Vermont Avenue, N.W.
Washington, D.C. 20005

also

7400 Skokie Boulevard
Skokie, Illinois 60077

American Society for Clinical Pathologists (ASCP)
1101 Vermont Avenue, N.W.
Washington, D.C. 20005
also
2100 West Harrison Street
Chicago, Illinois 60613

National Center for Allied Health Leadership
1 Dupont Circle, Suite 300
Washington, D.C. 20036

American Society of Allied Health Professions
1 Dupont Circle, Suite 300
Washington, D.C. 20036

American Chemical Society
1155 16th Street, N.W.
Washington, D.C. 20036

Joint Commission on Accreditation of Hospitals (JCAH)
645 North Michigan Avenue
Chicago, Illinois 60611

National Council for Radiation Protection (NCRP)
7910 Woodmont Avenue, Suite 1016
Bethesda, Maryland 20814

National Fire Protection Association (NFPA)
60 Batterymarch Street
Boston, Massachusetts 02110

National Safety Council (NSC)
444 North Michigan Avenue
Chicago, Illinois 60611

American Conference of Governmental Industrial Hygienists
  (ACGIH)
6500 Glenway Avenue, Building D-5
Cincinnati, Ohio 45211

American Hospital Association (AHA)
840 North Lake Shore Drive
Chicago, Illinois 60611
(Journal—*Hospitals*, Journal of the American Hospital Association)

American Industrial Hygiene Association (AIHA)
25711 Southfield Road

Southfield, Michigan, 48075
(Journal—*American Industrial Hygiene Association Journal;*
66 S. Miller Road; Akron, Ohio 44313)

American Medical Association (AMA)
Division of Scientific Activities
Department of Environmental, Public, and Occupational Health
535 North Dearborn Street
Chicago, Illinois 60610
(Journal—Journal of the American Medical Association, *Archives of Environmental Health*)

American Occupational Medical Association (AOMA)
150 North Wacker Drive
Chicago, Illinois 60606
(Journal—*Journal of Occupational Medicine;* P.O. Box 247;
Downers Grove, Illinois 60515)

National Academy of Sciences
Committee on Hazardous Substances in the Laboratory
2101 Constitution Avenue, N.W.
Washington, D.C. 20418

American Association of Blood Banks
National Office, Suite 600
1117 North 19th Street
Arlington, Virginia 22209

Clinical Laboratory Managers Association
23341 North Milwaukee Avenue
Half Day, Illinois 60069

American Medical Technologists
710 Higgins Road
Park Ridge, Illinois 60068

GOVERNMENT AGENCIES

National Institute for Occupational Safety and Health (NIOSH)
Office of Technical Publications
Robert A. Taft Laboratories
4676 Columbia Parkway
Cincinnati, Ohio 45226

U.S. Department of Labor
Occupational Safety and Health Administration (OSHA)
200 Constitution Avenue, N.W.
Washington, D.C. 20210

U.S. Government Printing Office (GPO)
Superintendent of Documents
Washington, D.C. 20402

U.S. Nuclear Regulatory Commission (NRC)
1717 H Street, N.W.
Washington, D.C. 20555

Centers for Disease Control (CDC)
1600 Clifton Road, N.E.
Atlanta, Georgia 30333

U.S. Environmental Protection Agency (EPA)
401 M Street, S.W.
Washington, D.C. 20460

National Institutes of Health (NIH)
9000 Rockville Pike
Bethesda, Maryland 20205

State and local health departments provide valuable sources of safety information and requirements.

INFORMATION ABOUT GASES

Matheson Specialty Gases
932 Paterson Plank Road
East Rutherford, New Jersey 07073

Union Carbide Corporation
Linde Division
308 Harper Drive
Moorestown, New Jersey 08057

SAFETY COURSES

J. T. Baker Chemical Company
Office of Safety Training
222 Red School Lane
Phillipsburg, New Jersey 08865

Government Institutes, Inc.
966 Hungerford Drive #24
Rockville, Maryland 20850

Norman V. Steere and Associates, Inc.
140 Melbourne Avenue, S.E.
Minneapolis, Minnesota 55414

National Cancer Institute
Office of Research Safety
National Institutes of Health
Bethesda, Maryland 20205

Centers for Disease Control
Laboratory and Training Division
Bureau of Laboratories
Atlanta, Georgia 30333

National Institute for Occupational Safety and Health
Training and Manpower Development
Robert A. Taft Laboratory
4676 Columbia Parkway
Cincinnati, Ohio 45226

TAPES AND PUBLICATIONS ON LABORATORY SAFETY

Slide-Cassette Tapes on Laboratory Safety
National Cancer Institute
Office of Research Safety
Bethesda, Maryland 20014

Order Desk
National Audiovisual Center (GSA)
Washington, D.C. 20409

Training and Information Resources
Division of Safety
Building 13, Room 2E43
National Institutes of Health
Bethesda, Maryland 20205

LIBRARIES

The National Library of Medicine
8600 Rockville Pike
Bethesda, Maryland 20209
(301-656-4000)

The Library of Congress
Washington, D.C.
(202-287-5000)

OSHA Technical Data Center
200 Constitution Avenue, N.W.
Washington, D.C. 20210
(202-523-6441)

SCIENTIFIC SUPPLY CATALOGS CONTAINING SAFETY EQUIPMENT

Safety Equipment for Science and Industry
Lab Safety Supply
P.O. Box 1368
Janesville, Wisconsin

Reagents and Laboratory Products
J. T. Baker Chemical Company
Phillipsburg, New Jersey 08865

Best's Safety Directory
AM Best Company
Oldwick, New Jersey 08858

Fisher Safety Manual
Fisher Scientific
711 Forbes Avenue
Pittsburgh, Pennsylvania 15219

Scientific Products
American Hospital Supply
American Scientific Products Division
1210 Wankegan Road
McGaw Park, Illinois

Thomas Scientific Apparatus Catalog
Arthur H. Thomas Company
Philadelphia, Pennsylvania

Bibliography

Acquired immune deficiency syndrome (AIDS): Precautions for clinical and laboratory staff. CDC Morbidity and Mortality Weekly Report 31, No. 43, 1982

American Chemical Society: RCRA and Laboratories. Washington, Department of Public Affairs, 1983

American Chemical Society: Safety in Academic Chemistry Laboratories, 3rd ed. Washington, American Chemical Society, 1979

Bests Safety Directory 1980. Oldwick, NJ, A. M. Best Company, 1979

Bond RG, Michaelsen GS, DeRoos RL: Environmental Health and Safety in Health Care Facilities. New York, Macmillan, 1973

Carlson J: Guidelines for Laboratory Safety for Medical Technologists, Policies and Procedures. Skokie, College of American Pathologists, 1976

Catalog 80: Reagents and Laboratory Products. Phillipsburg, NJ, J. T. Baker Chemical Company, 1980

College of American Pathologists' Laboratory Checklist. Skokie, College of American Pathologists, 1983

Fabian JT (ed): Chemistry Safety Monograph. Calgary, Canada, Calgary Board of Education, 1977

Flury PA, Deluca K: Environmental Health and Safety in the Hospital Laboratory. Springfield, IL Charles C Thomas, 1978

Halper RH, Foster HS: Laboratory Regulation Manual. Washington, Aspen Systems Corp, 1976

Heal AV, Miale JB, Weill CV: A previously unrecognized laboratory hazard: Hepatitis B antigen-positive control and diagnostic sera. Am J Clin Pathol 59:681–687, 1973

Henry RJ et al: Safety in the Clinical Laboratory. Van Nuys, BioScience Enterprises, 1976

Hepatitis B: A Review of Immunoprophylaxis and the Disease. Selected Reports from the Literature. West Point, PA, Merck, Sharp and Dohme, 1982.

Inhorn L: Quality Assurance Practices for Health Laboratories. Washington, American Public Health Association, 1978

Inspector's Manual for Accreditation of Medical Laboratories. Skokie, College of American Pathologists, 1980

Johnson JW, Stern EL et al: Aerosol production associated with clinical laboratory procedures. Am J Clin Pathol 29:591–599, 1974

Joint Commission on Accreditation of Hospitals: Accreditation Manual for Hospitals 1980. Chicago, Joint Commission on Accreditation of Hospitals, 1979

Krugman S: The newly licensed hepatitis B vaccine: Characteristics and indications for use. JAMA 247:2012–2015, 1982

Laboratories in Health-Related Institutions 1980 NFPA 56C. Boston, National Fire Protection Association, 1980

A Laboratory Safety Guide. The California Association of Public Health Laboratory Directors, 1980

Lathrop JK (ed): Life Safety Code Handbook NFPA 101, 2nd ed. Boston, National Fire Protection Association, 1981

Lennette EH, Schmidt NJ: Safety precautions for performing tests for hepatitis-associated "Australia" antigen and antibodies. Am J Clin Pathol 57:526–530, 1972

Manufacturing Chemists Association: Guide for Safety in the Chemical Laboratory, 2nd ed. New York, Van Nostrand Rheinhold, 1972

McKinnon GP: Fire Protection Handbook, 15th ed. Boston, National Fire Protection Association, 1981

McKusick BC: Prudent practices for handling hazardous chemicals in laboratories. Science 211:777–780, 1981

National Hazards Control Institute: Hazardous Materials Safety Seminar. Stanton, NJ, Starson Corporation, 1978

National Research Council: Prudent Practices for Handling Hazardous Chemicals in Laboratories. Washington, National Academy Press, 1981

Needlesticks Take High Toll. The Draw Sheet, University of Virginia, 1981, 30.

O'Neill GJ: Comment: A novel idea for communicating health and safety data. Chem Eng News 27, 1982

Pike RM: Laboratory-associated infections: Summary and analysis of 392 cases. Health Lab Sci 13:105–114, 1976

Radiation—A Fact of Life. Vienna, International Atomic Energy Agency, 1979

Richardson JH, Barkley WE (eds): Draft: Biosafety in Microbiological and Biomedical Laboratories. Washington, U.S. Department of Health and Human Services, 1983

Roach GC: Laboratory Safety: Principles for Personal Practice. Houston, American Society for Medical Technology, 1976

Safe Handling of Toxic and Hazardous Chemicals and Biologicals Product Catalog. Janesville, WI, Lab Safety Supply Company, 1981

Safety Committee: Safety Handbook. Fairbanks, University of Alaska, 1977

Special Issue. Laboratory Safety. Laboratory Medicine, 1980

Standards for Accreditation of Medical Laboratories. Skokie, College of American Pathologists, 1983

Stanley PE (ed): CRC Handbook of Hospital Safety. Cleveland, Chemical Rubber Company, 1981

Steere NV (ed): CRC Handbook of Laboratory Safety, 2nd ed. Cleveland, Chemical Rubber Company, 1971

Straub CP: CRC Handbook of Environmental Control. Cleveland, Chemical Rubber Company, 1975

The Health Hazard Evaluation Program of the National Institute for Occupational Safety and Health. Federal Register 37, No. 215, 1972

U.S. Code of Federal Regulations: General Domestic License for By-Product Material, Section 31.11, 10CFR31

U.S. Congress: Occupational Safety and Health Act of 1970. P.L. 91-596, 91st Congress, 1970

U.S. Department of Health, Education and Welfare, Center for Disease Control: Classification of Etiologic Agents on the Basis of Hazard, 1976

U.S. Department of Health, Education and Welfare, Center for Disease Control: Controlling Infections, Aerosols in the Lab. CDC Lab Update 78-37, 1978

U.S. Department of Health, Education and Welfare, Center for Disease Control: Health and Safety Guide for Hospitals. DHEW NIOSH 78–150, 1978

U.S. Department of Health, Education and Welfare, Center for Disease Control: Laboratory Safety at the Center for Disease Control. CDC 79–8118, 1979

U.S. Department of Health and Human Services, Center for Disease Control: Proposed Biosafety Guidelines for Biomedical Laboratories.

U.S. Department of Health, Education and Welfare, Center for Disease Control: Isolation Techniques for Use in Hospitals, 2nd ed. HEW Pub. 78–8314, 1975

U.S. Department of Health, Education and Welfare, National Institutes of Health: Biohazards Safety Guide, 1974

U.S. Department of Health, Education and Welfare, National Institutes of Health: Laboratory Safety Monograph: A Supplement to the NIH Guidelines for Recombinant DNA Research, 1979

U.S. Department of Health, Education and Welfare, National Institutes of Health: The National Institutes of Health Radiation Safety Guide. (NIH) 79–18, 1979

U.S. Department of Health and Human Services, Health Services Administration: Safe Practices: Vol. 1, Clinical Laboratories; Vol. 2, Hospitals and Health Care Facilities, 1978

U.S. Department of Labor, Occupational Safety and Health Administration: All About OSHA. OSHA 2056, 1980

U.S. Department of Labor, Occupational Safety and Health Administration: OSHA General Industry Standards (29CFR1910). OSHA 2206, 1978

U.S. Department of Labor, Occupational Safety and Health Administration: Recordkeeping Requirements Under the Occupational Safety and Health Act of 1970, 1978

U.S. Environmental Protection Agency: Draft Manual for Infectious Waste Management. U.S. EPA-SW957, 1982

Williams SV, Huff JC: Epidemic viral hepatitis, type B, in hospital personnel. Am J Med 57:904–911, 1974

Yesus YW: Post-transfusion hepatitis—update. Lab Med 12:703–706, 1981

Index

299